Philosophical Issues in Nursing

Also by Steven D. Edwards

Nursing Ethics: A Principle-based Approach (1996)
Externalism in the Philosophy of Mind (1994)
Relativism, Conceptual Schemes and Categorial Frameworks (1990)

Philosophical Issues in Nursing

Edited by

Steven D. Edwards
RMN, BA (hons), MPhil, PhD

MACMILLAN

First published 1998 by
MACMILLAN PRESS LTD
Houndmills, Basingstoke, Hampshire RG21 6XS
and London
Companies and representatives
throughout the world

ISBN 978-0-333-67210-5   ISBN 978-1-349-14235-4 (eBook)
DOI 10.1007/978-1-349-14235-4

A catalogue record for this book is available
from the British Library.

10 9 8 7 6 5 4 3 2 1
07 06 05 04 03 02 01 00 99 98

Editing and origination by
Aardvark Editorial, Mendham, Suffolk

CONTENTS

Keith Cash

RGN, RMN, BA(HONS), MSc, PhD

Occupation: Professor of Nursing, Faculty of Health and Social Care, Leeds Metropolitan University.

Recent Publications: Cash K. et al. *The Preparation of Sick Children's Nurses to Care for Children in the Community* (London: ENB, 1995). Benner and expertise in nursing: a critique, *International Journal of Nursing Studies*, **32**(6): 527–34, 1996. Social epistemology, gender and nursing theory, *International Journal of Nursing Studies*, **34**(2): 137–43, 1997.

Paul J. Dawson

RPN, BA(HONS), MA

Occupation: Research nurse, Psychiatric Nursing Research Institute, Royal Park Hospital, Melbourne, Australia.

Recent Publications: The impact of biological psychiatry on psychiatric nursing, *Journal of Psychosocial Nursing*, **34**(8): 28–33, 1996. In defence of the middle ground, *Journal of Advanced Nursing*, **19**: 1015–23, 1994. Philosophy, biology, and mental disorder, *Journal of Advanced Nursing*, **20**: 587–90, 1995. Contra biology: a polemic, *Journal of Advanced Nursing*, **20**: 1094–103, 1995.

Steven D. Edwards

RMN, BA(HONS), MPHIL, PhD

Occupation: Lecturer, Centre for Philosophy and Health Care, University of Wales, Swansea.

Recent Publications: *Externalism in the Philosophy of Mind* (Aldershot: Avebury, 1994). *Nursing Ethics, A Principle-based Approach* (London: Macmillan, 1996). What is philosophy of nursing?, *Journal of Advanced Nursing*, **25**: 1089–93, 1997.

Janet Holt
RGN, RM, ADM, RNT, PGDiPE, BA(HONS), MPHIL

Occupation: Lecturer, School of Healthcare Studies, University of Leeds.

Recent Publications: Ethics, Law and Nursing (co-authored) (Manchester: Manchester University Press, 1995). Screening and the perfect baby, in Frith, L. (ed.) *Midwifery Ethics* (London: Butterworth-Heineman, 1996).

Stephen Horrocks
RMN, RGN, BA(HONS), MPHIL (PHD CANDIDATE)

Occupation: Senior Lecturer in Mental Health Nursing, Department of Nursing, University of Salford.

Trevor Hussey
BA(HONS), MA, DPHIL

Occupation: Senior Lecturer in Philosophy, Buckinghamshire College of Higher Education.

Recent Publications: Nursing ethics and project 2000, *Journal of Advanced Nursing*, **15**: 1377–82, 1990. Nursing ethics and codes of professional conduct, *Nursing Ethics*, **3**(3): 250–8, 1996. Efficiency and health, *Nursing Ethics*, **4**(3): 181–90, 1997.

Edward P.R. Lepper
BA(HONS)

Occupation: Lecturer in Philosophy, Buckinghamshire College of Higher Education.

Recent Publications: What's wrong with diversity?, *Proceedings of Consensus in Bioethics* conference, University of Central Lancashire, 1996.

Joan Liaschenko
RN, MA, MS, PHD

Occupation: Assistant Professor, School of Nursing, University of Wisconsin, Milwaukee, USA.

Recent Publications: Artificial personhood: nursing ethics in a medical world, *Nursing Ethics* **2**(3): 186–96, 1995. The ethics in the work of acting for patients, *Advances* *in Nursing Science*, **18**(2): 1–12, 1995. Knowing the patient?, in Thorne, S. and Hayes, V. (eds) *Nursing Praxis: Knowledge and Action*, pp. 23–38 (Thousand Oaks, CA: Sage, 1997). The moral geography of home care, *Advances in Nursing Science*, **17**(2): 18–26, 1994.

Philip J. Ross
BA(HONS), PHD

Occupation: Lecturer, Faculty of Social, Health, Environmental and Life Sciences, University College of Ripon and York St John.

Recent Publications: *De-privatising Morality* (Aldershot: Avebury, 1994). Utility, subjectivism and moral ontology, *Journal of Applied Philosophy*, **11**(2): 189–99, 1994.

Simon Woods
RGN, BA(HONS) (PHD CANDIDATE)

Occupation: Macmillan Lecturer in Cancer Nursing, University of Liverpool.

Recent Publications: Cancer care and the moral implications of altered appearance, in de Beaufort I., Hilhorst, M. and Holm, S. (eds) *In the Eye of the Beholder, Ethics and Medical Change of Appearance*, pp. 197–205 (Copenhagen: Scandinavian University Press, 1996).

Introduction

Steven D. Edwards

A glance at the major journals of nursing research and scholarship reveals that, increasingly, nurses are turning to philosophy and to philosophers in their efforts to provide secure theoretical foundations for nursing theory and practice. The present volume provides further evidence of the existence of that attempt and gives an indication of its character. All of the contributors are involved in nurse education, all have qualifications in either nursing, philosophy, or both, and all have a serious research interest in philosophical aspects of nursing.

There is no doubt that philosophy of nursing is, as yet, a young discipline. There are few canonical works or 'standard texts'. Indeed, there are only a handful of book-length studies. Any attempt to acknowledge the pioneers of the subject would have to recognise the work of Professor Patricia Benner (for example, 1984, 1994; Benner and Wrubel, 1989), the efforts of Professor June Kikuchi (for example, Kikuchi and Simmons, 1992) in the Institute for Philosophical Nursing Research in the University of Alberta, and also the work of Rogers (1970), Watson (1979) and Parse (1981). In the United Kingdom, a recent book by Reed and Ground (1997) has attempted to set out the relations between philosophy and nursing in a way which, perhaps, is more systematic than has been achieved hitherto.

This book is a further articulation of the rich connections between philosophy and nursing. It is evident that the areas of interest of the contributors, within philosophy of nursing, are varied. However, common themes emerge, for example, regarding the understanding of the relationship between the mind and the body, and the status of what has come to be described as nursing knowledge.

But what is philosophy of nursing? I have tried to answer this question in more detail elsewhere (Edwards, 1997), but it is plausible to suppose that analysis of the concepts that are fundamental to nursing

1

comprises one of the tasks of philosophy of nursing. Consistent with that claim, many of the papers in this volume involve such analysis. The book includes philosophical examinations of concepts such as knowledge, holism and the self, all of which are plainly fundamental to nursing theory and practice. For example, with specific reference to the concept of the self, severe physical trauma (for example, severe burns), chronic illness and mental health problems are each plausibly regarded as having a deep effect upon self-identity.

In Stephen Horrocks's paper, the application of philosophical thought to the nursing curriculum is undertaken. Also, in what follows, more general issues relating to the nature and status of nursing are investigated. Janet Holt's paper is critical of much of what passes for 'nursing theory'. She points out that such theories are frequently described as 'philosophies' (Marriner-Tomey, 1994). Yet, she suggests, they do not stem from rigorous philosophical analysis. Part of the explanation of this, Holt argues, stems from the fact that many contributors to the nursing literature do not have a clear conception of just what philosophical enquiry is.

Roughly speaking, there are four main areas of philosophical enquiry: ontology, epistemology, value-enquiry and logic. Crudely, ontology involves investigation into the nature of things: what is it to exist?; what is a particular item – is it an object?; if so, of what sort is it?; what is the distinction between particular things and the kinds of which they are members?; what distinguishes one thing from another thing? – these are questions that fall within the realm of ontology. Some of the papers in this volume examine ontological questions. For example, Edward Lepper conducts an ontological enquiry into the nature of mind. He wonders what the 'best' theory of mind for nursing might be and what criteria should be employed in order to determine this. Paul Dawson enquires into the nature of the self; again, this is an ontological enquiry. Trevor Hussey's paper also conducts an ontological enquiry into the nature of change. He indicates how analyses of change in the natural world can be shown to have a fruitful application to the realm of ideas and theories. Simon Woods' paper on holism also embraces ontological concerns. As he suggests, one of the ways in which holism has come to be described is as an ontological claim relating to the constitution of things. Holism is commonly taken as claiming that things are 'more than' or 'greater than' simply the sum of their constituent parts. Hence, patients and clients are 'more than' simply the sum of their constituent body-parts.[1]

The second main category of philosophical enquiry identified above is epistemology. Again crudely, the focus of epistemology lies in the concept of knowledge. Within the province of epistemological enquiry, one asks questions such as the following: what is the difference, if any, between knowing something and merely believing it?; if we think there is a difference, we suppose there to be some distinction between belief and knowledge: what might this be? Also, within the province of epistemological enquiry, one may raise questions concerning whether there are differing types of knowledge, such as knowledge of how to perform certain skills, and knowledge that certain facts are true. Furthermore, one may enquire into the question of whether there are special sources of knowledge. For example, does the access one has to one's own thoughts bring with it a degree of certainty about what it is one is thinking or feeling? Of the papers in this collection, Joan Liaschenko's paper seems to be engaged in an epistemological enquiry. She wonders why such great credence is accorded to propositional knowledge, or 'knowledge that' something is the case. She suggests that one of the reasons why 'nursing knowledge' is often not recognised as such is due to the fact that much of it is 'hidden', hidden in the sense that much of it involves 'knowing how' and this category of knowledge is not accorded due status. It is characteristic of knowing how that it cannot be made explicit; it resists description in sets of rules or sets of sentences. The status accorded to 'knowing that' thus partly generates a view in which nursing knowledge has little status – in so far as it resists summary description. Moreover, she provides a fascinating explanation of the reasons for the status accorded to knowledge that can be made explicit. She undertakes this by examining a key transition in the history of medicine: a transition from an era in which the workings of the body are 'hidden' from view – the era of what she terms the 'closed body' – to an era in which these workings are deemed open to view – the era of the 'open body'.

Keith Cash is engaged in a related project in his contribution. He suggests that one way to conceive of nursing is as a 'practice'. It is characteristic of practices that those within them share criteria for what constitutes a problem within the practice, and also for what a solution to the problem must look like. Hence, members of a practice typically agree on the kinds of problem that require answers and on the methods that are most appropriately implemented in order to answer such problems. In my own contribution, the suitability for nursing of positivist method is discussed. Since positivism can be described as a method for finding out about the world, this chapter also lies within the province of epistemology.

The third area of philosophical enquiry mentioned above is that of value-enquiry, the main components of which are ethics and aesthetics. These are properly described as part of the province of value-enquiry since they seem to concern judgements that are value judgements. The suggestion is that moral judgements express the values of the judger. A judgment that action A is right or good indicates that the person making the judgement values actions of type A. Similarly with aesthetic judgements: a judgement that a work of art A is better than another work of art B seems to imply that A is valued more highly than B. In the present collection, there are no papers concerned with aesthetics, and, perhaps, only Philip Ross's paper is concerned explicitly with ethics. The reason for this is that there seem to be a considerable number of books already available on the subject of nursing ethics. Also, part of the rationale for the present volume is to try to show how other areas of philosophical enquiry can be applied fruitfully to nursing.

The fourth and final area of philosophy to be mentioned here is that of logic. In outline, this involves an enquiry into argumentation itself, into the relations of implication that hold between the patterns of claims that comprise arguments. The focus of logic is not on the details of specific arguments or sets of claims, but rather on the form of such arguments. None of the papers in this collection is a paper devoted to the study of logic. Although, of course, all involve argumentation, none of the papers is devoted to the study of argumentation itself.

The above four-fold division of the concerns of philosophy is, at most, a rough and ready classification. There is much debate concerning the separability of the four areas. This is especially true of the relationship between ontology and epistemology. For example, a criticism of positivism is that it 'tailors' ontology to fit its epistemology, so only those things which can be found to exist by the application of the positivist method have a legitimate claim to 'really' exist. However, for our purposes, the four-fold division just discussed provides a useful schematic outline of the types of philosophical inquiry. However, readers should bear in mind that, in actual philosophical enquiry, it is frequently impossible to adhere rigidly to such divisions.

Readers will notice that each of the papers in the following collection is preceded by a brief summary. These summaries are written by the editor and are intended to signal the main concerns and steps occurring in the paper. They are intended as rough guides for the reader.

I would like to close this introduction by thanking the contributors for their enthusiastic participation in this project. Thanks are due, also, to Richenda Milton-Thompson of Macmillan for encouraging the idea of a book such as this in the very early stages of its production.

NOTES

1. For the sake of simplicity, I have chosen to use the term 'ontology' here in preference to the term 'metaphysics'. Strictly speaking, although the enquiries of Edward Lepper and Paul Dawson are legitimately described as ontological, Trevor Hussey's enquiry is metaphysical: it is more general than the kind of existence-questions discussed by Edward Lepper and Paul Dawson.

REFERENCES

Benner, P. (1984) *From Novice to Expert* (Menlo Park, CA: Addison-Wesley).

Benner, P. (ed.) (1994) *Interpretive Phenomenology* (London: Sage).

Benner, P. and Wrubel, J. (1989) *The Primacy of Caring* (Menlo Park, CA: Addison-Wesley).

Edwards, S.D. (1997) What is philosophy of nursing?, *Journal of Advanced Nursing*, **25**: 1089–93.

Kikuchi, J.F. and Simmons, H. (eds) (1992) *Philosophic Inquiry in Nursing* (London: Sage).

Marriner-Tomey, A. (1994) *Nursing Theorists and Their Work*, 3rd edn (St Louis: CV Mosby).

Parse, R.R. (1981) *Man-Living-Health: A Theory of Nursing* (New York: John Wiley).

Reed, J. and Ground, I. (1997) *Philosophy for Nursing* (London: Edward Arnold).

Rogers, M. (1970) *An Introduction to the Theoretical Basis of Nursing* (Philadelphia: FA Davis).

Watson, J. (1979) *Nursing: The Philosophy and Science of Caring* (Boulder, CO: Colorado University Press).

Part I

NURSING PRACTICE AND KNOWLEDGE

CHAPTER ONE

The shift from the closed to the open body – ramifications for nursing testimony

EDITOR'S INTRODUCTION

Joan Liaschenko argues that much nursing knowledge is not recognised as such – is not legitimated. Part of the explanation for this lies in the fact that much of it is hidden from view, or is simply not accorded due status or cannot be made explicit. The medical enterprise prohibits the legitimation of knowledge that is not open to view.

Joan Liaschenko's explanation of this phenomenon draws attention to a key transition in the history of medicine, one captured in the three illustrations that accompany her chapter. The transition is from a view in which the inner workings of the human body are understood to be hidden, to a view in which its workings are held to be open to view.

This 'objectification' of the human body has had several consequences. One such consequence, as noted, is the emphasis upon objective data, but another is the objectification of patients themselves, manifested in the focus on patients as 'diseases' rather than as ill persons. Hence, the shift that Liaschenko discusses, if she is correct, has had a deep effect upon the nature of the relationship between physicians and patients.

Furthermore, the shift from the closed to the open body brings it about that key components of nursing knowledge only find expression amongst nurses themselves. It is expressed in the '"let's get real" language that nurses share among themselves in the private space of shift reports' (see p. 18). This 'let's get real' language, a potentially rich source of nurse testimony, passes unnoticed outside the profession; it is not accorded the status of knowledge, it is not legitimated.

Joan Liaschenko argues, finally, that the shift in medicine to the open body generates two conceptions of nursing. In one, nurses are portrayed simply as friendly faces. In the other, nurses are portrayed as technicians comfortable with the complex technology of ICU. Her chapter shows the profound inadequacy of each of these two conceptions of nursing.

The shift from the closed to the open body – ramifications for nursing testimony

Joan Liaschenko

It is commonly understood that nursing work involves watching patients on a variety of dimensions and reporting those observations to someone, usually a member of the medical profession. This dual process of observing and telling can be considered as a kind of testimony, one of the three sources of knowledge within Anglo-American epistemology (Coady, 1992, pp. 3–24; Code, 1995, pp. 64–74). Yet the testimony of nursing is differentially received. While some nursing knowledge (and, by extension, nursing work) is highly visible within the culture, retaining legitimacy and commanding a certain authority, large portions are invisible and silenced. In this chapter, I suggest that the nursing testimony deemed legitimate, is so because it is a direct extension of scientific medicine. This is to say that when nurses are the eyes and ears of the physician, they see, hear and report what can be contained within the discourse of scientific medicine.

Nurses know, however, much more than merely a certain portion of scientific medicine. A large measure of the power of scientific medicine is that it can be represented, that is, made visible to the public eye. The significance of this in contemporary society is that only what can be represented counts as knowledge and what does not count as knowledge is either readily dismissed, ignored or, worse still, not even seen, regardless of how important it might be. This chapter explores one reason for this power of representation within scientific medicine.

In the first section of the chapter, I discuss four kinds of knowledge that involve witnessing and telling: knowledge of therapeutic effectiveness, knowledge of how to get things done, knowledge of patient experience and knowledge of the limits of medicine. Only one of these, however, is received as knowledge by the dominant discourse of scientific medicine. The next section discusses the notion of representation and is followed by an examination of the shift in medical knowledge from the closed body to the open body, a shift that lends itself more readily to representation. In the final section, I raise some challenges that this representation poses for nursing.

TESTIMONY

There are two reasons for exploring nursing knowledge and its legitimation from the framework of testimony. First, testimony is similar to the idea of advocacy, with which nurses are quite familiar. However, whereas advocacy emphasises speaking to someone on behalf of a patient, testimony underscores the idea of bearing witness to the event about which one then speaks. Also, while advocacy is most commonly understood as having a moral sense, it is also understood as doing work that connects patient and services for the purpose of influencing some patient outcome (Jacques, 1993). Even when restricting our use to the former sense, unless one is going to speak blindly, advocacy also requires knowing something about the goods of human life as well as how they relate to the best interests of the particular patient.

In recent theoretical literature, formal testimony is seen as involving some matter (in dispute) about which someone deemed competent gives evidence to some audience (Coady, 1992, pp. 25–53). Testimony involves bearing witness as the means of access to knowledge as well as the telling of that knowledge. The idea of competence is concerned to answer two questions: what counts as evidence?, and who is competent to give it? To give testimony is to present oral evidence; it is to speak the truth of some phenomena. What is considered to be true, however, may differ between communities of knowers.

For example, the present paper had its origins in an empirical study that sought to understand the ethical experience of practising nurses (Liaschenko, 1993). For these nurses, advocacy was central to their practice. Interestingly, the situations in which they advocated for patients involved conflicting epistemologies, most often between nursing and medicine. Nurses advocated for patients in those situations where their knowledge of the patient and situation conflicted with that of the physicians. The process of advocacy was an attempt to have physicians come to see and know differently. Because testimony is a richer notion emphasising what and how something is known, I conceptualised the moral work of advocacy as testimony.

The second reason for exploring nursing knowledge as testimony is that testimony is concerned with the subjectivity of the knower. As numerous philosophers have pointed out, most of us depend on the knowledge obtained by others most of the time. This is true even in the 'hard sciences' like physics. For example, Hardwig (1985, pp. 345–8) notes that not every experiment reported in physics journals is repeated in order to verify the results. When evaluating knowledge from a second-hand source, the believability of the speaker becomes a major factor. Questions of evidence and who is competent to give it involve assumptions concerning the trustworthiness of the speaker (Baier, 1986; Fricker, 1987; Hardwig, 1991; Coady, 1992, pp. 46–7). As feminist philosopher Lorraine Code points out, in mainstream epistemology 'pride of place' is given 'to the cognitive products of the "exact sciences"' (Code, 1995, p. xii). In other words, the only legitimate knowledge is scientific knowledge, and the trustworthiness of the speaker depends in large measure on whether or not the speaker speaks from within the scientific canon. These matters are of singular import to feminist epistemologists because the knowledge that people (often women) have about how the world is and works that is obtained from local practices and oral traditions is discounted as knowledge. Because they do not speak from the dominant discourse of scientific knowledge, their knowledge lacks authority or, even worse, is discounted as knowledge in the first place.

Nursing is a boundary discipline. It operates within and at the margins of a number of disciplines, each of which has its own knowledge base. Clearly, a major portion of nursing work shares the knowledge of scientific medicine. This is obvious in such things as physical assessment, judgement about when to initiate therapeutics and monitoring for therapeutic effectiveness. However, nursing work also involves forms of knowledge that are not scientific, such as knowing how to get things done within a given institution, knowledge of patient experience and, oddly enough, knowledge of the limits of scientific medicine. Using the ideas of formal testimony, some matter of import, competence, evidence and audience, I briefly consider these four examples of nursing knowledge about which nurses observe and speak to others. My aim is explication: I want to show how nursing knowledge is used by nurses and responded to by others.

Knowledge of therapeutic effectiveness

Monitoring patient responses to medical treatment is the most visible, well-defined and, perhaps, common understanding of nursing practice. With this type of knowledge, nursing's primary audience is medicine and the evidence is physiological or, in some cases, psychological. Nurses keep the sick body under surveillance through the lenses of scientific knowledge such as anatomy, physiology, mechanisms of disease, pharmacology and other therapeutic procedures. Bodies are observed, measured and assessed against some scientific norm, and therapeutics are commonly initiated by nurses – what is usually thought of as following orders. This work involves discrimination and judgement (Benner, 1984) and is not the mere reporting of information. In telling about the patient, nurses are making knowledge claims that they support with physiological or psychological evidence.

The competence of nurses to monitor the effectiveness of medical interventions is a very complex issue involving such factors as the division of labour, social status and power, gender issues and the regulatory bodies that oversee the respective practices. The competence of nurses to monitor medical therapeutics varies but is generally accepted. Such acceptability, however, is a historical process partially related to innovations in scientific medicine and technology. Work is handed down to those of lower status as it becomes routine (Hughes, 1993, p. 307). For example, Koenig (1988) found that one process in the routinisation of medical technology is to turn the actual use of it over to nurses. Although Koenig was not studying nursing competence, her work suggests that nurses are seen as competent as technology becomes routine. The association of nursing competence with monitoring by technology should not be confused, however, with the control of that technology. Nursing does not control the technology, neither its development nor its deployment.

In monitoring for therapeutic effectiveness, the nurse is the eyes and ears of scientific medicine. Present-day nurses actually talk of themselves in this way (Liaschenko, 1994), but this idea originated at a time when medicine was challenging nursing's legitimacy to share the therapeutic space at the bedside. Nurse historian O'Brien D'Antonio (1993) showed that nurses won the right to be at the bedside only by submitting their knowledge to the authority of physicians. Being the eyes and ears of medicine means that only certain aspects of reality can be seen and heard, and therefore afforded legitimacy, within this discourse. The knowledge that falls outside the parameters of scientific discourse is ignored, seen as trivial or denied as knowledge. It is this knowledge that concerns me in the remainder of this section.

Knowledge of how to get things done

Knowledge of how to get things done is not readily analysed through the concept of testimony. This kind of knowledge involves knowing how to get things done in very complex situations and environments. The knowledge I am referring to is not technical knowledge such as inserting a nasogastric tube or making an evaluation of side-effects from medication. Rather, the knowledge I have in mind is a matter of connecting the patient to resources; it is the sense of advocacy mentioned earlier. Such know-how is not a small matter in terms of skill or in terms of the significance to the well-being of patients. Health-care delivery systems in the United States are highly fragmented, often requiring patients to go to several places and providers for care. Indeed, this fragmentation of care is thought to be a moral harm by some nurses (Liaschenko, 1997). Navigating this geography of resources and services for patients is commonly thought of as the coordination of care and is critical to patient well-being. The knowledge involved is not merely one of the resources required but of how to access and deploy those resources within a temporal framework, the timeliness of which may mean a great deal in terms of alleviating patient suffering.

The audience to whom nurses might speak in making these connections can include a vast hierarchy and network of people and agencies, amongst them professional, governmental and community. The nurse's experience and effectiveness in arranging for resources are generally considered evidence that the nurse knows what she or he is doing, and competence is assumed by the organisational power structure. Yet I do not wish to give the impression that there is too much made about nursing competence in this arena. On the contrary, there is a taken-for-grantedness about these activities in an institution; in fact, they are invisible to the institutional power structure. These connecting activities are thought simply to happen and they are not identified as work.

In his study of nurses, Jacques, an organisational theorist, commented that while these activities and the related activities of conveying information to the appropriate people enable the institution to function, they are neither a 'core criteria for reward and advancement in organizational personnel systems' nor 'a source of power in organizational governance and decision making' (Jacques, 1993, p. 3).

The idea of invisible work is not new to nursing (Wolf, 1989; Liaschenko, 1997), and scholarship in the area corroborates that done by other scholars across different contexts (De Vault, 1991). What is particularly noteworthy is that institutional power structures, including scientific discourse, function in such a way as to prevent the people performing these connecting activities from considering them as work. This is true whether the people are women feeding their families (De Vault, 1991), female engineers keeping projects going through interpersonal work (Fletcher, 1994) or the nurses in Jacques' study.

Testimony involves speaking the truth about some phenomena. It requires a community of interlocutors (Felman and Laub, 1992; Liaschenko, 1995); it requires acknowledgement. Within health care, the public is shielded from how much of this kind of knowledge is necessary to their well-being; left undisputed is the illusion that they are well because of the miracles of scientific medicine. This is, of course, true, but it is only a partial truth. Jacques (personal communication, 1996) gives a very telling example. A nurse in his study spent approximately 2 hours trying to get pain medication increased for a post-surgical patient. She finally reached the physician and got the order increased. However, what is publicly represented to the world is that the physician ordered an increase in medication and the nurse followed the order. Completely invisible is, to borrow Murdoch's concept, the attentive gaze (Murdoch, 1985, p. 34) through which the patient's suffering is revealed, the knowledge involved in locating the physician and presenting the case, the time involved and the skill of attending to this while doing multiple things simultaneously. These activities have no status as work, they are not recognised as knowledge, and they cannot be spoken of in the giving of testimony.

Knowledge of patient experience

A third kind of knowledge in nursing practice is knowledge of patient experience. By this I mean to convey something different from the knowledge obtained as the eyes and ears of the physician. As the latter, the nurse's attention is framed by the parameters of what scientific medicine considers significant: that is, physiological or psychological data. People generally do not live their lives in the discourse of medicine. Rather, they live in the language of everyday life, in the places and temporal rhythms that make up that everyday life, connecting them to others and generating a history. Knowledge of patient experience requires a repositioning of the nurse so that her or his gaze moves from the body as an object of medical intervention to the body of someone living a life. Access to this knowledge requires an attentive gaze (Murdoch, 1985, p. 34) and heartfelt listening to the stories of disrupted lives. Through this gaze and this listening, practitioners come to know the meaning of therapeutic interventions for patients and can hear when enough is enough. They can see the significance of behaviours that practitioners so easily diagnose as non-compliance as well as other expressions of patient subjectivity (feelings and emotions) that can frustrate practitioners in the smooth execution of what is, for them, routine work (Hughes, 1993, p. 316).

Central to theoretical work in testimony is that there is some contested matter at stake, not a routine matter but a serious one, one significant to the life of the community as a whole. Conflicts between what is considered best by scientific medicine and what is considered best by the patient are not uncommon. Certainly, a patient's experience of her or his illness is anything but routine. Most nurses have a story in which they have spoken for a patient against some unwanted medical intervention or advocated for the patient to be seen and heard on her or his own terms. Speaking from the knowledge of patient experience on matters of import about which there is disagreement challenges prevailing medical wisdom and questions the legitimacy of scientific discourse as final authority. The competence of the nurse (and the patient) in this regard is highly questioned even though the evidence that the nurse (and the patient) gives is the patient's witnessing to her or his own suffering (Frank, 1995).

Medicine is not unconcerned with its treatment of patient experience as there is a small but very vocal discourse on the importance of attending to the patient's story; see, for example, Brody (1987) and Kleinman (1988). However, this is a minor chorus within scientific medicine, the main focus of which is not primarily patient care but rather research and technological innovation. It should be stressed that I am not talking here about individual physicians. Many physicians are committed to understanding their patients in this way. Rather, I am discussing the discourse of scientific medicine that fails to take account of the individual, experiencing patient.

Knowledge of the limits of medical science

Largely by witnessing the experience of patients, nurses recognise that medicine is not omnipotent. By this, I do not mean that medicine fails to cure on every occasion. On the contrary, I mean that the discourse of medicine fails to see that such an end is an illusion, the continued pursuit of which frequently causes great harm (Connors, 1980; Liaschenko, 1995). Nonetheless, nursing does not often speak to this; in fact, it has been claimed that nursing keeps the secrets of medicine (Alavi and Cattoni, 1995). There are many reasons for this silence, and a full exploration would take us beyond this chapter. One relevant to my point, however, is that scientific medicine does not have room for other insights. Nurses are silent on the limits of medicine because they occupy a very complex position in health care. As noted earlier, nursing is a boundary discipline, operating at the edges of competing epistemologies. Nurses operate both within the discourse of scientific medicine and outside it. The view from the periphery is different from that from the centre. It is the part nurses share with medicine, such as monitoring for therapeutic effectiveness, that grants them legitimate authority. However, as we have seen, nursing has eyes and ears for other things, and when nurses shift their gaze and voice, the discourse of scientific medicine cannot accommodate them; there is no more space.

Code's concept of rhetorical space is very relevant here. In her words:

> rhetorical spaces... are fictive but not fanciful or fixed locations, whose (tacit, rarely spoken) territorial imperatives structure and limit the kinds of utterances that can be voiced within them with a reasonable expectation of uptake and 'choral support': an expectation of being heard, understood, taken seriously. (1995, pp. ix–x)

The space of scientific medical reasoning is not structured to accommodate the visions of other gazes. Nurses do not have 'an expectation of being heard, understood, taken seriously' within medicine on certain issues, so their voice goes underground, so to speak. After failed attempts and sometimes no attempts to obtain the audience of medicine, they speak another language. It is the 'let's get real' language that nurses share among themselves in the private space of shift report (Liaschenko, 1993, p. 256) or other places where the matters of significance to patients and nurses can be spoken of and genuinely heard.

Thus far, I have attempted to show that, with the exception of the knowledge in monitoring for therapeutic effectiveness, the discourse of scientific medicine fails to legitimate the kinds of nursing knowledge that can be seen and heard from the rhetorical spaces of nursing work. In the next section, I explore one reason why this might be so. My suggestion is that, in stark contrast to medical knowledge, most of nursing knowledge cannot be readily represented.

REPRESENTATION OF WORK AND KNOWLEDGE

The notion of representation is a complicated one in contemporary thought (Rosenau, 1992, pp. 92–108), but I am using it in the rather straightforward sense of making something manifest (or visible), largely through some process of symbolisation. Recall the example of the post-surgical patient's need for pain medication. The physician's written order is a visible representation, a symbol of legally recognised authority to access prohibited drugs. Implicit in this representation of authority is the recognition that there is knowledge of pharmacology, physiology and so forth that 'stands behind' this order. This representation of authority and knowledge is understood within the larger culture; the order shows what doctors do. This may be even more clear in terms of visual images. Pictures of a surgical operation, or (indeed) even the incision and exposed organs, are understood by viewers. Such images convey that a great deal of skill and knowledge is involved in opening the human body. When we see such images, we know what a surgeon does. The same is the case with images from physicians and technical devices, for example, a computerised axial tomography (CAT) scanner. Even if the average viewer does not understand what the device is for and how it works, she or he knows, in some sense, what the physician is doing – trying to make one well. It is my contention that the ease of representing medical work and knowledge follows directly from the ability of scientific discourse to expose the inner workings of the human body. Great good has come from this but there have been significant losses as well. In the next section, I explore the shift from what can be termed 'the closed body' to what can be termed 'the open body'.

THE DISCOURSE OF SCIENTIFIC MEDICINE

In his book *The Birth of the Clinic*, Foucault traced the historical circumstances of modern medicine that wedded a way of seeing to a way of talking, which he conceptualised as the 'gaze' of medicine (Foucault, 1973, pp. ix–xix). For Foucault, structures of medical perception became linked to a certain language, in this case the language of the newly emerged science of the 1700s. Put simply, what could be seen by medical practitioners changed with how that knowledge was represented in the discourse of science. Consider the implications of Foucault's example in the shift in language from 'What is the matter with you?' to 'Where does it hurt?' (1973, p. xviii). Each of these questions sees different aspects of the sick body and allows for different answers, revealing stark differences in what can be known about the sick person as well as how the sick person is understood and subsequently treated. In asking, 'What is the matter with you?', the sick person is made a central actor in a dialogue, with a licence to tell his or her story as well as a certain authority to name. However, if we ask, 'Where does it hurt?', the answer points to a location in the body; the question does not solicit a story of a life lived.

Shifting from the first to the second question has been hugely successful for medicine. Advancing technology has enabled medicine to turn the body 'inside out' (that is, has made the inner workings of the body open to view), which has, in turn, advanced the development of therapeutics. These advances, however, make the sick person's story (by which I mean the narrative that connects the experience of sickness to the disruption of their everyday lives; Charmaz, 1991) less relevant. By turning the body inside out, medicine makes visible not only the body, but also its own knowledge. These advances have depended on the transformation of 'What is the matter with you?' to 'Where does it hurt?' In turn, this shift in medical perception and way of talking has altered the relationship between patient, physician and nurse. What follows are representations of the evolution of medical knowledge. These visual images tell a story of the changes in the gaze of medicine, from 'What is the matter with you?' to 'Where does it hurt?'

Representations of medical knowledge

The closed body

In Figure 1.1, we see the first drawing of anatomy known in the Western world, published in 1345 by the Italian physician Vigevano.[1] Vigevano was not the first to open the human body, however; that distinction belongs to his teacher, the physician Mundinus of Bologna, who did so in 1306. What is immediately striking about this illustration is the relationship between the anatomist and the dead person. van den Berg calls our attention to the fact that, although the incision has been made, we see nothing inside the body. Indeed, our gaze is directed towards the faces and the physical contact between them. Notice how the anatomist gazes rather tenderly at the eyes and face of the dead person. As van den Berg notes:

> The dead man is a human being, even if he is dead. He is not a corpse. Even less is he an anatomical specimen. He is a dead person and with this person the anatomist has an understanding. He talks to him, as it were; he consults with him. However we express it, there is a human contact. (1978, p. 70)

The anatomist cradles the body of the dead man, supporting him, as it were, against his own ambivalence of cutting. As van den Berg sees it, it is as if the anatomist does not really want to do this cutting, but he must. For his part, the dead man does not want this but submits to the inevitable.

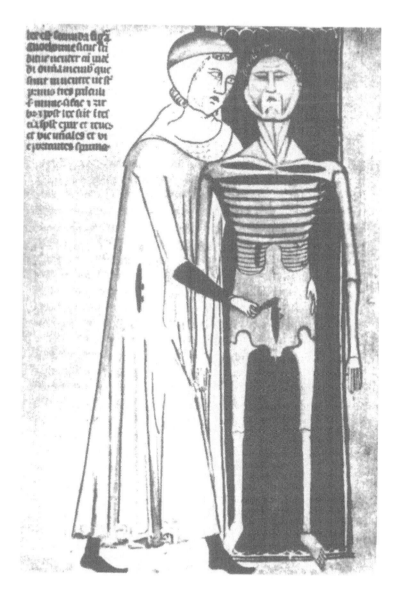

Figure 1.1 A 14th-century post-mortem examination

The text in the upper left hand corner of the drawing comprises medieval Latin words telling the reader what has been observed as a result of the incision:

> This is the second illustration, which shows how the belly is incised so that all parts within become visible. That is: the three layers of the abdominal wall: muscles, peritoneum serous membrane, then guts, spleen, liver, kidneys and urinal and seminal tract. (van den Berg, 1978, p. 71)

van den Berg points out the marked inconsistency between what the words tell us we see and what we actually see. All that we see is blood; we can not see into the body at all. In his view, blood is a warning that the body does have an inside. When we see blood following a cut, 'we are seeing the limit of what is visible "within" the unopened body' (p. 72). van den Berg calls this the closed body. As a closed body, the dead person is not yet an 'object' of medical science, a machine to be fixed.

What is really so striking is the recognition between the anatomist and the dead person. The eyes of the anatomist reveal a knowledge of recognition: he knows the other, not intimately as one might know a family member, neighbour or member of one's community, but as a member of the larger human community of which the anatomist clearly sees himself as belonging. This is important because in this recognition is the awareness that the anatomist, too, will become ill and die. Such an understanding is critical to the anatomist's ability to bear witness to the suffering of the other as 'testimony is inherently a process of facing loss' (Felman and Laub, 1992, p. 91). It is the recognition that death is one of the realities that all human communities confront (Nussbaum, 1988, p. 35). As viewers, we see this recognition in the eyes and posture of those depicted in it. The anatomist does not see the other as other but the other as himself. The techniques of success that will come from the newly opened body have not yet altered the relationship between person and disease, and person and practitioner (Hawkins, 1984).

The open body

Within 200 years, increases in our knowledge of the workings of the human body meant that the body was, quite literally, turned inside out. In 1543 the Flemish physician Vesalius, recognised as the father of modern anatomy, published *De corporis humani fabrica*, from which Figure 1.2 was originally taken. Immediately, we see a change in the relationship between the anatomist and the dead person. van den Berg draws our attention to the fact that the dead person is less human than the one subjected to Vigevano's knife. Vesalius's dead person is faceless and the identity made even more ambiguous by the artist's representation – having already been turned into an object. There is, for example, no obvious gender. While the dead person is large with well-developed muscles, which would suggest a male, the breast tissue seems too rounded for a man. Also, the hair is confusing: the length suggests that of a woman and, although it could be that of a man, the hair of the male anatomist is short. In contrast to Vigevano's closed body, this body is clearly open. There is no blood to warn that the body has an inside, and the gaze of the viewer is taken beyond the surface of the lived body directly into the recesses of the previously invisible body. The workings of the body are rendered machine-like.

Perhaps most telling is the anatomist himself. No longer is he gazing apologetically, tenderly at the dead person; he is not even looking at her or him. His gaze is directed towards an audience to whom he appears confident and, perhaps, even triumphant. To van den Berg, the anatomist has a look of 'benevolent firmness' (1978, p. 77). Look at the position of Vesalius's arms: they are nearly in the same position as Vigevano's but, while the latter cradles a human being, Vesalius holds forth a dissection. In 200 years, the gaze of medicine has transformed the human being into specimen. 'What is the matter with you?' is becoming 'Where does it hurt?'

I am intrigued with van den Berg's description of the anatomist's expression as one of 'benevolent firmness'. His only explicit explanation of this phrase is that Vesalius 'wants to show something to the reader' (1978, p. 77). But why does this showing demand benevolent firmness? Does the benevolence suggest an understanding, an empathy with the reader in the realisation that we lose something in a knowledge system that turns the body inside out? Is the firmness a support, an extension of Vigevano's inevitability? Or is it coercion, a not unsubtle force pushing us where we do not wish to go? van den Berg does not raise these questions explicitly but, rather, implicitly in talking about the period between Vigevano and Vesalius. During that time, much dissection was carried out but little was observed, and Galen's medicine was left intact. Only Da Vinci observed, but his work went unnoticed until after the time of Vesalius. Did we really need 200 years to be able to 'see' the open body? If so, why?

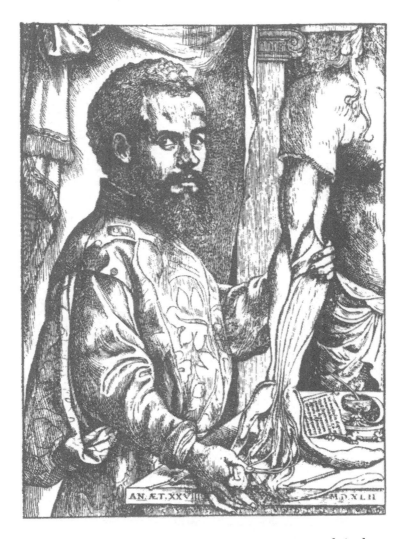

Figure 1.2   This is an anonymous engraving of Andreas
Vesalius (1514–1564), dissecting the forearm of a corpse

Modern scientific medicine

The third representation of medical knowledge comes 300 years later in the late 19th century. This is *The Agnew Clinic*[2] by the American painter, Thomas Eakins (Figure 1.3). This painting conveys the work and social organisation of medical knowledge. We see not only medical interventions on the open body, but also the various relationships constituting health care. The amphitheatre is centre stage and a fitting metaphor for the dramatic benefits of the emerging medical techniques. Three junior physicians or students are performing surgery, their focus reflecting a concentrated attention on specific parts of the body. If one were to draw a line from their eyes to the patient, one can see that their line of vision is centered on an important but nonetheless limited view. The attending physician, on the other hand, directs his gaze outward and over his subordinates; he is not looking at the patient and is removed from any direct contact with her. The physician has garnered a powerful audience in the social organisation of medical knowledge into a profession. He is both supervising the work and transmitting knowledge.

Notice the depiction of action. The animated intenseness of the attending physician and the precision of the students' movements are nearly palpable. Contrast this with the nurse whose quiet stance does not suggest work. She is positioned to see all four physicians. She is standing at attention in a state of readiness to be routed on command for some supply, some requirement necessary to the surgery, to medical work. Although her attentiveness and readiness cannot readily be represented as work, all is not lost on the artist. Eakins does show us the gaze of the nurse. In fact, we are drawn to the quiet intensity of her attentiveness. If we were to sketch a line from her eyes to the patient, we would find her gaze, like the anatomist of the closed body, directly fixed on the face, the most profound aspect of our identity, our individuality. We recognise and are recognised by others, largely through our faces. She is concerned with the woman as a closed body, and it is this gaze that keeps the patient central.

SOME CHALLENGES FOR THE GAZE OF NURSING

The gaze of nursing embraces all of the knowledges I have discussed, but most important to keeping the patient central are the ones that cannot be represented and are not recognized. *The Agnew Clinic* shows the nurse without an audience, without authority. She cannot

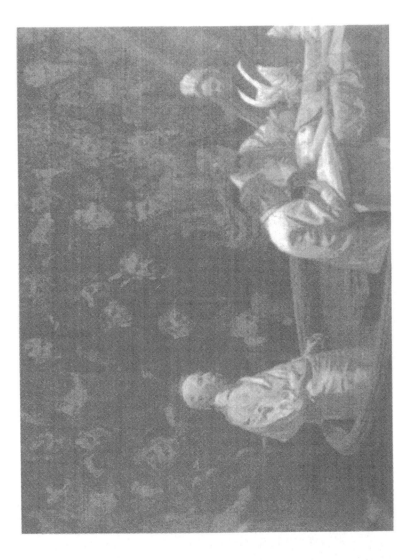

Figure 1.3 *The Agnew Clinic* by Thomas Eakins, 1889

order or even request things from the physician; she does not have a history of experimental science and discoveries that opened the human body, thereby legitimising her voice. She does not control the intervention techniques of the open body. Nonetheless, Eakins placed her historically and we are led to wonder how nursing knowledge and work are represented now, a hundred years later.

I would suggest that there are two ways, one being that of the emotional caretaker documented so well by Smith (1992). Smith found that much advertising depicts nurses in what are generally thought of as caring roles. They are talking to patients, holding their hands, listening attentively and supporting patients as they walk. In contrast to those of their medical colleagues, these images do not suggest that special knowledge, indeed any knowledge, is involved in this work. The knowledge of how to get things done, of patient experience, of the limits of medical science cannot be conveyed in these images.

In direct contrast, the second way depicts nurses as technical masters and therefore knowledgeable. Space does not permit a reproduction of the example I have in mind, but it is also an advertisement, one which appeared in a major scholarly nursing journal. The advertisement, released by a prominent US school of nursing, was aimed at recruiting doctoral students. In the advertisment, three white-coated individuals are comparing notes as they view some monitoring device. No patient is in the picture. These two images seem to be the only way we currently have of representing nursing knowledge and *neither* accurately does so.

Smith's findings show that nursing occupies a certain rhetorical space, a gendered space characterised largely by women doing women's work. As such, nurses are doing what is natural, speaking the unspeakable and 'knowing' what is not considered to be knowledge. Our important, multiple skills are not rendered any more visible by this representation of nursing. However, it is equally deceiving to conceive of nurses only as the eyes and ears of scientific medicine. If we limit ourselves to such a conception, we run the very serious risk of losing the proper gaze of nursing precisely because the discourse of the open body is highly restrictive in what it can accommodate.

Resolving this dilemma poses a challenge, the solution of which has overlapping political, moral and epistemological aspects. Since my aim in this chapter has been explication, I can only mention these. Politically, a solution to the problem will require working towards building a community of knowers of both the open and the closed body, even as we resist the silencing of our non-scientific knowledge. Epistemologically, it will require theorising about the connecting work that nursing does, what Fletcher terms 'relational practices' (1994, pp. 1–3, 78–134). Such theorising will move beyond the limits of the purely interpersonal to include the structural aspects of our work and knowledge. Finally, the moral aspect will involve a critique of our epistemologies – what is knowledge for?; who controls it?; how do we come by it?[3]

NOTES

1. Figures 1.1 and 1.2 are taken from *Medical Power and Medical Ethics* by J. H. van den Berg, New York: WW Norton, 1978. My discussion of these two figures draws heavily on Dr van den Berg's illustrative analysis, which I have paraphrased in some detail. This work of Dr van den Berg's has been indispensable to my own thinking, and I am grateful to him.
2. I gratefully acknowledge the University of Pennsylvania School of Medicine for permission to reprint Figure 1.3, *The Agnew Clinic* by Thomas Eakins, 1889.
3. This work was based on ideas developed from an earlier project funded by the National Institute of Nursing Research (#F31 NRO6836), the Graduate School and the Century Club of the University of California, San Francisco, and a PEO Scholar's Award. The author wishes to thank Dr Joanne Hall, Dr Patricia Stevens and, in particular, Dr Roy Jacques and the editor, Dr Steven Edwards, for fruitful discussion.

REFERENCES

Alavi, C. and Cattoni, J. (1995) 'Good nurse, bad nurse...', *Journal of Advanced Nursing*, **21**: 344–9.
Baier, A. (1986) Trust and antitrust, *Ethics*, **96**: 231–60.
Benner, P. (1984) *From Novice to Expert: Excellence and Power in Clinical Nursing Practice* (Menlo Park, CA: Addison-Wesley).
Benner, P. and Wrubel, J. (1989) *The Primacy of Caring: Stress and Coping in Health and Illness* (Menlo Park, CA: Addison-Wesley).
Brody, H. (1987) *Stories of Sickness* (New Haven: Yale University Press).
Charmaz, K. (1991) *Good Days, Bad Days: The Self in Chronic Illness and Time* (New Brunswick, NJ: Rutgers University Press).
Coady, C.A.J. (1992) *Testimony* (Oxford: Clarendon Press).
Code, L. (1995) *Rhetorical Spaces: Essays on Gendered Locations* (London: Routledge).
Connors, D.D. (1980) Sickness unto death: medicine as mythic, necrophilic and iatrogenic, *Advances in Nursing Science*, **2**(3): 39–51.
De Vault, M.L. (1991) *Feeding the Family: The Social Organization of Caring and Gendered Work* (Chicago: University of Chicago Press).

Felman, S. and Laub, D. (1992) *Testimony: Crisis of Witnessing in Literature, Psychoanalysis, and History* (New York: Routledge).

Fletcher, J. (1994) Toward a theory of relational practice in organizations: a feminist reconstruction of 'real work', unpublished doctoral dissertation, School of Management, Boston University.

Foucault, M. (1973, trans. A.M. Sheridan Smith) *The Birth of the Clinic: An Archaeology of Medical Perception*, (New York: Vintage Books).

Frank, A.W. (1995) *The Wounded Storyteller: Body, Illness, and Ethics* (Chicago: University of Chicago Press).

Fricker, E. (1987) The epistemology of testimony, *Proceedings of the Aristotelian Society*, **61**: 57–83.

Hardwig, J. (1985) Epistemic dependence, *Journal of Philosophy*, **82**(7): 335–49.

Hardwig, J. (1991) The role of trust in knowledge, *Journal of Philosophy*, **88**(12): 693–708.

Hawkins, A. (1984) Two pathographies: a study in illness and literature, *Journal of Medicine and Philosophy*, **9**(3): 231–52.

Hughes, E.C. (1993) *The Sociological Eye* (New Brunswick, NJ: Transaction Publishers).

Jacques, R. (1993) Untheorized dimensions of caring work: caring as a structural practice and caring as a way of seeing, *Nursing Administration Quarterly*, **17**(2): 1–10.

Kaplan Daniels, A. (1987) Invisible work, *Social Problems*, **34**(5): 403–15.

Kleinman, A. (1988) *The Illness Narratives: Suffering, Healing, and the Human Condition* (New York: Basic Books).

Koenig, B. (1988) The technological imperative in medical practice: the social creation of a 'routine' treatment, in Lock, M. and Gordon, D. (eds) *Biomedicine Examined*, pp. 465–96 (Dordrecht: Kluwer Academic).

Liaschenko, J. (1993) Faithful to the good: morality and philosophy in nursing practice, unpublished doctoral dissertation, University of California, San Francisco.

Liaschenko, J. (1994) The moral geography of home care, *Advances in Nursing Science*, **17**(2): 16–26.

Liaschenko, J. (1995) Artificial personhood: nursing ethics in a medical world, *Nursing Ethics*, **2**(3): 185–96.

Liaschenko, J. (1997) Ethics and the geography of the nurse–patient relationship: spatial vulnerabilities and gendered space, *Scholarly Inquiry For Nursing Practice: An International Journal*, **11**(1), 45–59.

Murdoch, I. (1985) *The Sovereignty of Good* (London: ARK Paperbacks).

Nussbaum, M.C. (1988) Non-relative virtues: an Aristotelian approach, in French, P.A., Uehling, T.E. and Wettstein, H.K. (eds) *Midwest Studies in Philosophy*, volume XIII, pp. 32–53 (Notre Dame: University of Notre Dame Press).

O'Brien D'Antonio, P. (1993) The legacy of domesticity: nursing in early nineteenth-century America, *Nursing History Review*, **1**: 229–46.

Rosenau, P.M. (1992) *Post-modernism and the Social Sciences: Insights, Inroads, and Intrusions* (Princeton, NJ: Princeton University Press).

Smith, P. (1992) *The Emotional Labour of Nursing* (Basingstoke: Macmillan).
van den Berg, J.H. (1978) *Medical Power and Medical Ethics* (New York: WW Norton).
Welbourne, M. (1979) The transmission of knowledge, *Philosophical Quarterly*, **29**: 1–9.
Wolf, Z.R. (1989) Uncovering the hidden work of nursing, *Nursing and Health Care*, **10**: 462–7.

CHAPTER TWO

Traditions and practice – nursing theory and political philosophy

EDITOR'S INTRODUCTION

Keith Cash points out that nursing theories tacitly presuppose or stipulate some conception of what nursing is. His claim is that such theories have not yet been successful and that this is, in part, due to their omitting to consider appropriately the question of what nursing is. Cash proposes that one fruitful way of conceiving of nursing is as a practice in the sense of that term explicated by MacIntyre (1985). In MacIntyre's account, the identities of practices are anchored in their histories, in tradition. Furthermore, it is argued that practices have certain characteristic, unifying features. For example, they embody a shared conception of what 'good practice' within the practice consists of. Hence, participants in a practice can be expected to share certain values and recognise certain virtues. Also, ways of resolving disputes within the practice (what Cash terms 'argumentation conditions') are characteristically recognised. So members of a unified practice can be expected to apply similar criteria for the recognition of problems within the practice and also for the resolution of such problems. Agreement in argumentation conditions means that members of a practice will be in a position to reach agreement concerning when a problem has arisen within the practice, how a problem can be posed and what will count as its resolution. Thus, a unified practice has resources within it which can resolve problems.

Cash suggests that arriving at an agreed set of argumentation conditions within nursing (where this is considered as a practice in MacIntyre's sense) has proved elusive, hence the problems in arriving at a widely agreed theory of nursing. Cash identifies a number of reasons why it has proved problematic to provide a unifying account of nursing as a practice; for example, he locates problems posed for nursing by the medical and managerial traditions. However, he closes the chapter with a

proposal of his own: that the practice of nursing can be unified by refer-
ence to certain virtues that have traditionally been fundamental to
nursing. Readers can judge for themselves whether they find his
proposals compelling.

Readers may care to note certain common themes between Keith
Cash's chapter and that of Joan Liaschenko. Both are preoccupied with
the nature of nursing and nursing knowledge. Also, it appears, both are
prepared to sanction an account of nursing in which knowledge and truth
are 'relativised' to practices or contexts. Trevor Hussey's chapter, which
follows Cash's, also seems sympathetic to a view in which practices
(specifically, that of scientific enquiry) do not discover truths but merely
move from adherence to one theory, to another 'better' theory.

Traditions and practice – nursing theory and political philosophy

Keith Cash

Nursing theory is an attempt to organise and describe a number of practices and, by so doing, to delineate the domains of practice that are proper to nursing. By implication, this means that theoreticians are involved in the task of defining nursing. The theoretical bases of nursing theorists are numerous and include those taken from the fields of positivism (such as Roy, Johnson and Orem) phenomenology (Benner) and existentialism, broadly defined (Parse and Watson). Despite an imposing edifice of nursing models, there is little evidence that they have made a contribution to the development of nursing practice (Cash, 1992). This chapter will examine some ideas that contribute to an understanding of this failure.

Contrary to the essentially modernist project of nursing theory, it has been argued by philosophers such as MacIntyre (1985), and nursing theorists such as Benner (1996), that there is a primacy of tradition in the way that practices are to be understood. Some sense of tradition is important if there is to be an articulation of the meaning of practices. This chapter will examine accounts of tradition and the ways in which they relate to nursing practices. Specifically, the implications of accounts of tradition for the way in which nursing theory has been developed will be elaborated. The main proposal of this chapter is that it is not possible to understand a project such as nursing without recourse to an idea of tradition; however, as will be seen, there are substantial theoretical problems associated with using that concept.

As Benner has pointed out, it is necessary to distinguish between traditions and traditionalism (1996). The latter is the uncritical following of historically established practices where the authority of the practice is its historical continuity; the former is more complex. The claim is that practices cannot be understood except in the context of the tradition that they define. There are several theories of the relationship of tradition and practice, each of which has different implications for the development of nursing theory. I will examine two of these theories to determine what is useful in the idea of tradition and which idea is the strongest. I will argue that the idea of tradition is useful for providing a context for argumentation about nursing but that the concept has some implicit difficulties. These are related to the issues of whose tradition one is referring to, who determines the tradition, how boundaries between traditions are to be determined and, crucially, the relationship of tradition to power. However, despite these difficulties, the attempt to describe and argue about the traditions of nursing can provide an intellectual focus for nursing that nursing theories do not provide because, in many ways, they make important assumptions about precisely what those traditions are or should be.

PRACTICES AND TRADITION

We can begin by establishing the case that there is a difference between scientific and practical knowledge that justifies introducing an external factor such as tradition into a discussion of practices. For example, Kenny (1992) argues that the difference between scientific and practical knowledge relates to the concept of truth. If I make a statement of fact, it is either true or untrue. If, however, I make a statement related to action, what might be seen as a correct statement could then lead to unacceptable results. For example, it could be that if I decide to cut someone with a knife, what distinguishes that from a criminal assault is that I am trying to debrade a wound, and my act is undertaken within the context of a whole collection of legal and professional rules and customs. The act is given its meaning by the context in which it takes place. The rules, therefore, are contextually dependent in a way a scientific law would not be. If I drop a scalpel and it falls to the floor, it will do so at a predictable rate of acceleration, that of gravity, no matter where on earth I do so. Thus, there appears to be a significant difference between scientific and practical reasoning. The former is basically 'acontextual' while the latter is context-dependent.

Our next question, then, concerns the nature of the context that gives meaning to practical decision-making. Individual propositions have meaning within a particular context. The context that provides this meaning can be interpreted in several ways. The first is the Cartesian sense that other propositions give meaning to an expression (for example a formal expression), an example of this being a computer programme. Another is in the positivist sense that propositions are meaningful only if they are verifiable; otherwise, they are literally nonsense. There is also a school of thought which argues that the concept of tradition is central to the understanding of the contextual nature of practical reasoning, 'practical reasoning' referring to reasoning that leads to an action. In this chapter, I wish to consider two main views: those of the Aristotelians in the person of MacIntyre, and the Heideggerians such as Benner. There are other important thinkers in this area, for example, conservative thinkers such as Oakeshott, but the main arguments in relation to tradition can be examined by concentrating on MacIntyre and Benner. Their positions entail some notion of tradition where tradition is conceived of as a particular cocktail of practices that gives meaning to the activities of the practitioners within that tradition. Each of these positions has a different explanation of the way in which this cocktail is constituted.

MacINTYRE'S POSITION

One influential account of what this means is that of MacIntyre's Aristotelian idea of virtues and their emergence from practice. By a practice he means:

> any coherent or complex form of socially established human activity through which goods internal to that form of activity are realised in the course of trying to achieve those standards of excellence which are appropriate to... that form of activity. (1985, p. 187)

A practice also involves standards of excellence and obedience to rules in addition to the achievement of goods. As he says:

> to enter into a practice is to accept the authority of those standards and the inadequacy of my own performance as judged by them. (1985, p. 190)

The virtues are understood as dispositions that sustain practices. For example, try to imagine the practices of nursing being undertaken without the virtues of compassion, justice or courage. These are among the virtues whose presence or absence determines good from bad nursing care. MacIntyre also makes a distinction between internal and external goods. He gives the example of a chess player who cares mainly about the fame and financial rewards that emerge from success at the game rather than caring about the game itself. MacIntyre says that, in such a case, the player could have achieved these ends by doing almost anything else. He does not achieve the internal goods of chess, the excellence that is specific to chess and the satisfaction that follows from this.

As MacIntyre describes it, a tradition is 'then a historically extended socially embodied argument, and an argument precisely in fact about the goods which constitute that tradition' (1985, p. 222). In that sense, traditions are moral orders that are historically constituted and have three characteristics that can be distinguished:

1. They can be a way of shaping or transmitting practices over time.
2. They can be a way of understanding the worth and importance of practices.
3. They can be moral or religious, economic, aesthetic or geographical.

What are the strengths of this model of tradition as it applies to nursing? The first is that it puts nursing practice firmly into the realm of the social. The individual nurse is part of a discipline, a set of practices, that has a history. It stresses that a practice is never merely a set of technical skills but rather that these skills serve certain goods and ends. Because nursing practices are social they have a history and a tradition.

However, for each individual, the practice of the virtues can only be understood in terms of the personal narrative of that individual. The reason for this is that the actions of individuals are to be understood by recourse to this narrative. Narratives are an expression of, amongst other things, the traditions that have informed them. For example, many nurses work in areas where there is some personal risk to themselves, frequently with patients who have a stigma associated with their illness because of the risk to themselves perceived (correctly or incorrectly) by the general public.

One example of this is the case of nurses who work with people who have infectious diseases, some of which have low survival probabilities or are currently incurable, and for which no vaccines exist (diseases such as Lasa and Ebola fevers and HIV). This area of work is interesting because the statistical probabilities of incurring infection can be calculated, but the only way of understanding those probabilities, of making sense of the risk that they exemplify, is by looking at the personal narratives of the nurses who work in those areas and at how they construct risk. For example, the chance of seroconversion after a needlestab injury from a needle that has just injected a person with AIDS is about 1 in 200 (Cash, 1995); the chance of receiving a needlestab depends on the incidence of these on one's unit. How these odds are interpreted is a function of how a particular individual constructs risk, how that statistical probability is weighed and judged.

For example, I once interviewed a Charge Nurse with a long experience in this area of work, who had a deep understanding of the risks

that were present in it and the sense that one had to have some vocation to work with this group of patients. In other words, there were
some 'goods' internal to this work that made sense of the risks one
took. The term that encapsulates the meaning of this sort of narrative
is 'vocation' (although this is now seen as rather old-fashioned,
perhaps owing to its religious associations). The idea of vocation is
more than a question of attitude but rather indicates a moral and
social position; a person pursuing a vocation feels a certain dedication
and fitness to perform the relevant role.

These last remarks suggest that, in order to gain the inner goods of a
practice, some personal risk has to be taken. It is difficult to see any
practices where abstaining from risk could lead to the gaining of the
relevant 'internal' goods. For people to evaluate probabilistic risks in
an altruistic way requires some sense of belonging to a community
with a tradition that enables them to construct a personal narrative
making sense of this risk. The division between internal and external
goods also has implications for the drive of some nurses for professionalisation. Status, power and financial rewards are external goods that
can be obtained from other activities; they bear little relationship to the
internal goods of nursing. Similarly, managerial virtues of control and
manipulation, and the virtues of nursing, seem at first sight to be
incompatible. They raise two different practices and two different traditions – and thus two sets of possibly competing virtues.

BENNER AND A HEIDEGGERIAN POSITION

A further influential description of practices is that offered by Benner
(1984). She argues that there is a hermeneutical project necessary to
make explicit the practices of nursing. The philosophical basis for her
claim lies in the work of Heidegger, as interpreted by Dreyfus and
Dreyfus (1985). The idea of tradition is central to this approach. Practices are not propositional in character, that is, they cannot be reduced
to a series of statements (such as computer code). Rather, they are
given their meaning by the tacit background in which they are
embedded; hence, the description of practices is a hermeneutical
activity (a matter involving the interpretation of, and immersement in,
such practices). I have argued elsewhere that there are some fundamental problems with Benner's approach (Cash, 1995) apart from the
issue of tradition. In terms of the latter (that is, the description of the
practice) there are further difficulties, not least because there is no
extensive description of what would constitute the appropriate tradi-

tion or traditions. In Benner's discussion, the concept of tradition is under-defined. It is possible to discern two distinct interpretations of her position.

The first is what we can call the concept of the naïve tradition. Here, there is either an uncritical acceptance of the tradition or considerable authority inherent in the tradition. In other words, the tradition is apparent, unproblematic and to be followed. In the next sense, the tradition is to made clear by the hermeneutical investigator. She examines current practices and produces a description of the practices and their tacit background. In a weak interpretation of her position, this description is the end product. However, in a stronger interpretation, the description of the practices uncovered by the hermeneutical inquirer provides a basis on which to argue the nature of the practices. Interpreted in either the strong or weak way, Benner uses a model that is taken from elsewhere (the Dreyfus model of skill acquisition, which is seen as a universal characteristic of people) and locates her description of clinical practice within that. However, of course, the idea of skill and skill taxonomies is highly appropriate to a managerial tradition of examining practice. In this tradition, the idea of the manipulation of resources and the mixing of resources to maximise profitability is seen as central. The 'good manager' is one with the appropriate skill mix of employees, one that maximises output and minimises costs. Benner's project is therefore firmly located within a tradition that is, paradoxically given Heidegger's work on technology, compatible with the technocratic ethos of managerialism.

Benner, however, contends that there is an argument in favour of additions to a tradition, and to the argumentation conditions of a tradition, in order to introduce a critical element into it. She holds out (Benner, 1996) for a critical theoretical and feminist approach to the description of practice. Here, she recruits elements that are not part of the tradition of nursing, for example, Marxism (in the form of critical theory) and feminism, neither of which have been a significant strand of the culture or curricula of nursing (see Cash, 1997). The claim, therefore, that these epistemologies should be used to explicate the tradition of nursing seems to have the following flaws.

1. It assumes that the argumentation conditions for adjudicating between arguments do not exist in the traditions of nursing but should rather be taken from other traditions, for example, Marxist sociology in the case of critical theory, the technological in the case of systems theory.

2. Related to the above is the issue of who selects the 'alien' epistemology to be recruited in explication of the tradition of nursing. For example, critical theory is unlikely to be accepted as a basis for practice in most clinical areas because it is a theory of Marxist origin, which, if used reasonably, has substantial implications for the power structures in society. It is a liberatory epistemology in this interpretation. If we are to explicate the practice of nursing and therefore the tradition(s) of nursing by recourse to this theory, we are either arguing that this should become the theoretical core of nursing, with all that this implies, or claiming that it is a means of understanding nursing in the way in which, say, we could use functionalism to understand a primitive society. In the former, we act as epistemological insiders, in the latter as outsiders. Now this has an interesting implication for the idea of tradition? If I am both an insider and an outsider, what is the tradition? Does the positioning of one person cause the tradition to alter? Is it possible to create new argumentation conditions for the tradition?

Our discussion of MacIntyre's and Benner's derived notion of tradition and its application to the description of nursing practice raises several issues. These include: what precisely is meant by the idea of tradition?, who decides what the tradition is?, and how can we decide between different traditions?

WHAT IS MEANT BY A TRADITION?

There are three elements of a tradition that are accepted in different formulations by various theorists who use the notion:

1. The tradition consists of patterns of practices that are combined in a manner that is bounded. The tradition and its interpretation is therefore a closed or partially closed body.

2. Certain practices are legitimate. There is some sense of the interdependency of practices. Each practice is not a separate entity but rather there are links between the practices.

3. There can be some legal constructions of the tradition, especially in the case of professions.

There is no doubt that the idea of tradition, even in its loosest sense, implies some argument or dominant interpretation about what constitutes that tradition. It is also the case that, when two traditions come into contact, there is the possibility of conflict and a process of argumentation that is not solely intellectual, but also related to the relative resources controlled by the respective traditions. Nursing has, of course, existed since the 19th century in tandem with medicine and was intellectually in thrall to that discipline for much of the time. Nursing carved out its territory in the United Kingdom because resources vital to the activities of medicine were controlled by nursing. The budgets held by Directors of Nursing, and the educational budgets held by the statutory regulatory bodies, meant that nurses might be educated in the medical model. However, there was considerable 'slippage'. Where the will to do so was present, nurses were able to control the 'caring side' of health care. This has changed in recent years with the growth of general management and the removal of nursing budgets. It now means that, if general managers appreciate the contribution of nurses, there is the possibility of development. If, however, they do not, there is an emphasis on skills as discrete units to be manipulated in the most cost-effective manner. There is, therefore, a conflict between two sets of virtues – those of cost–benefit managerialism and those of nursing care. The resolution of that conflict is related to the nature of the argumentation conditions that prevail both within and between the two distinct traditions.

ARGUMENTATION CONDITIONS

I have previously mentioned the notion of the argumentation conditions that exist in nursing. Argumentation conditions are those generally accepted ways of arguing within a tradition that enable the tradition to develop, they are the internal standards of justification. These standards allow a tradition to solve its outstanding problems when inconsistencies arise or responses to new external situations are necessary. For ideas of tradition to amount to more than simply that traditions involve the uncritical and unchanging transmission of authority, some description of how they can change is necessary. This is why MacIntyre's notion of argumentation conditions is useful.

For example, the use of critical theory, undifferentiated feminist theory, existentialism, systems theory and so on involves the appeal to theories that have no currency in the tradition of nursing. The appeal to these external sources is a sign of a lack of confidence in, or an absence of, internally based argumentation conditions. If it is argued that the deference to externally validated epistemologies is a part of the tradition of nursing, it follows from the discussion above that the nursing tradition is a weak and perhaps an ultimately doomed one. Similarly, part of the project of developing nursing theory involved an attempt to state explicitly the criteria for adopting a theory (Fawcett, 1980). This strategy worked both to create argumentation conditions and to state what they would be. This has not succeeded because there is no critical consensus that one can find in the nursing literature concerning what such a theory would look like. There are many authoritative statements but no critical literature where argumentation conditions are worked through.

This has very practical consequences for the establishment of a nursing voice in the current health-care system. For example, in many health services at the moment, there is the introduction of health-care workers, of varying degrees of skill, whose role is controlled by managers rather than by interaction between professional regulatory bodies and managers. Concepts such as that of 'vocation' are not part of the discourse relating to the health-care worker, unlike in nursing, in which there is a history featuring that concept. However, it is also the case that the idea of vocation can be interpreted in several ways within nursing. For example, it could be seen as the expression of a moral position of unselfishness from which acts of nursing are undertaken from a moral position rather than a desire for monetary gain. However, it could also be interpreted as the expression of the subjugation of female ambitions by the transference of the qualities of mothering to the clinical situation. However, the issue for a tradition is not that disputes arise within it, for, unless the strong authoritarian definition of tradition is the one accepted, all traditions will have internal disputes. The question is rather what conditions are necessary to resolve the dispute, in fact what the conditions are that allow the dispute to occur in the first place.

This is the next characteristic of argumentation conditions: they explain how a dispute has arisen and not hitherto been solved. The issue of unskilled health-care workers is interesting here because the issue has not been solved by nursing. Many of the changes to the means of implementing health care have been instigated by non-nurse managers. Managerialism embodies a set of virtues different from that embodied in nursing. Nursing is not primarily about the control and manipulation of resources, but it is true that, historically, many nursing roles have had substantial managerial elements. These include, for example, the Charge Nurse with her team of trained and untrained staff, and the Director of Nursing with the nursing workforce budget. There is, therefore, a dispute in nursing concerning the management of care, and this dispute has not been resolved.

DECIDING BETWEEN TWO TRADITIONS

An important question, especially owing to the situation in which nursing presently finds itself, is how it is possible to select between traditions. This question has two elements: The first is what the internal conditions are for selecting between competing interpretations of the tradition, and the second concerns the external conditions for the selection of a tradition.

The first issue has been discussed in the section on argumentation conditions. For the second, some general principles seem to apply. First, there is clearly a battle when traditions start to compete. The victory of a particular tradition is related to the 'epistemic status' carried by its members and the resources they control. Such resources may be economic or epistemological, for example, the control of academic journals or the control of certain university departments – these are arenas where ideas are legitimised. For nursing, I have suggested above that the competing traditions are managerialism and medicine. In both cases, these control resources, although they, too, are in conflict with each other.

Furthermore, nursing has specific problems in terms of epistemic status because it is still predominantly a female occupation. The literature on the gendered basis of knowledge is now copious (Cash, 1997). Coupled with this is the problem that nursing does not engage the outside world in the discussion of the virtues of nursing and thus engage others in a debate about them. Much of the theoretical literature in nursing is arcane, not only to outsiders but also to insiders, and this is a reflection of the lack of clarity concerning the argumentation conditions in nursing.

WHAT ARE THE TRADITIONS OF NURSING?

Nurses practice in a tradition and the virtues of the good nurse are defined within that tradition. Without the idea that our narrative is grounded in some sort of grander narrative, we become disorientated. Values and virtues are historically constructed. History consists in argument about narratives that are considered to be important. It is impossible to enter into discussion about what nursing is without addressing where it came from. For example, an important motif in nursing history is that Nightingale went to the Crimea to look after a despised group – the soldiery – and did so by the application of sensible public and clinical health measures. She did not establish the nursing order (a religious term) to look after the rich. In that sense, she was acting congruently with those religious orders which had gone before her. Another thing she did was to organise the order for the benefit of middle-class women who wished to escape the home. Since women were excluded from trade and the universities were closed to women until the late 19th century, and with the need to maintain a safe sexual distance between women and men, the nursing order was 'gendered' (Witz, 1992).

The historical tradition of nursing can be seen to have several strands, including that of the church, the military and the legacy of Nightingale in institutionalising nursing by invoking the state and formalising the requirements to be a nurse. This formal element is the one that was exported and which provided the model for other countries. It can be argued, therefore, that nursing emerged in some way from a common core and that this has provided a large element of the nursing tradition. For many years, this tradition was passed on by the socialisation of new nurses using a quasi-military and religious model. The virtues of nursing were passed on in an authoritarian and patriarchal culture in which nurses were not encouraged to take a critical stand and in which deviants were expelled from the profession. Within this tradition, the idea of selfless care was paramount in a way analogous to that of the mother or wife putting the interests of offspring and spouse first. In this model, the underlying virtues are related to the good nurse being the good woman, showing the womanly virtues of sacrifice and service. This is a model arguing that the relationship between doctor and nurse is analogous to that between male and female. The caring that nursing does is therefore as invisible, to use Oakley's term (Oakley, 1985), as is housework or the rearing of infants.

So we have two strands to the practice of nursing: on the one hand, the religious and military delivery of care, and on the other, the 19th century creation of nursing on the basis of gender in a patriarchal society. There are, therefore, two interlinked traditions. Female Charge Nurses in the United Kingdom are still called Sister and the term 'Matron' is being reintroduced in some hospitals to replace 'Director of Nursing'. However, the gendered nature of nursing is not historically the oldest. For example, Wright (Wright and Hearn, 1993) has written of the historical existence of male nursing orders such as the Alexian Order, which was founded in 1334 (Kaufman, 1978). The members of this Order nursed outsider groups such as plague victims and lepers; those who still exist today nurse the mentally ill and AIDS patients. Similarly, there were military nursing orders who cared for the sick and also fought in battle, a curious mixture, from the contemporary view, of the feminine and the masculine. Nursing, therefore, is not just, it appears, a gendered occupation but one that is linked to certain virtues. In the examples I have given, these virtues are both Christian and patriarchal.

In the above brief discussion regarding the traditions of nursing, I have pointed to a non-gendered tradition based upon the notion of nurses caring for groups that are in some way marginalised by society: the mentally ill, the elderly, the incurably ill and the homeless. To practice this nursing well requires the exercise of certain virtues, both moral and technical. The description and argument of what these virtues are, or should be, is the central contribution that an examination of the traditions of nursing can make. From the construction of the traditions that I have briefly given above, I would argue that these include a non-discriminatory stance, in fact a stance that looks to the neglected, the stigmatised and the dangerous as people of value who deserve good care. The desire to give the best care in the circumstances, the best care being that delivered on the best evidence, seems to require a nurse who is not motivated by the external goods of financial rewards. What is also apparent is that, in arguing for the sort of moral order that this implies, it is not sufficient to take the view of the Alexian brothers of the humility and invisibility of good works. Such a position means the ultimate extinction of these universal values by the pressures of the market; what we need is the political will of Nightingale and a debate about the virtues of nursing.

CONCLUSION

There are several ways of approaching the idea of tradition, some more useful than others. All involve a relationship between authority, either political or epistemic, or both, and practice. I have suggested that several traditions exist in nursing. What these traditions are is open to debate. However, there do not seem to be well-established argumentation conditions for deciding between them. This could be a reflection of the weakness of the intellectual tradition in nursing, in which case it is not inevitable that nursing will survive. As Giddens has pointed out:

> All disciplines have their fictive histories, all are imagined communities which invoke myths of the past as means of both charting their own internal development and unity, and also drawing boundaries between themselves and other neighbouring discipline. (1996, p. vii)

In that sense, the idea of tradition is useful, but the relationship of tradition with authority, especially for a (now) gendered occupation like nursing, always has to be salient. Nursing theory does not offer a solution because it confuses internal and external argumentation conditions. In other words, it generally tries to set up the argumentation conditions with reference to other dominant epistemologies. Those nursing theories that do not do this do not engage, except by appeals to authority, in a debate with competing traditions, especially medicine and managerialism. One cannot, therefore, escape talking about traditions, if one wishes to make sense of practices, but the debate over what that tradition is, and the authority that it holds, is very much a political one.

REFERENCES

Benner, P. (1984) *From Novice to Expert: Excellence and Power in Clinical Nursing Practice* (Menlo Park, CA: Addison-Wesley).

Benner, P. (1996) A response by P. Benner to K. Cash, Benner and expertise in nursing: a critique, *International Journal of Nursing Studies*, **33**(6), 669–74.

Cash, K. (1992) Formal models, tacit knowledge and expertise in psychiatric nursing, unpublished PhD thesis, University of Manchester, Manchester.

Cash, K. (1995) Benner and expertise: a critique, *International Journal of Nursing Studies*, **32**(6): 527–34.

Cash, K. (1997) Social epistemology, gender and nursing theory, *International Journal of Nursing Studies*, **34**(2): 137–43.

Dreyfus, H. and Dreyfus, S.E. (1985) *Mind Over Machine* (New York: Free Press).

Fawcett, J. (1980) A framework for analysis and evaluation of conceptual models of nursing, *Nurse Educator*, Nov–Dec: 10–13.

Giddens, A. (1996) *Politics, Sociology and Social Theory* (Oxford: Polity Press).

Kaufman, C. (1978) *History of the Alexian Brothers: Ministry of Healing*, vol. 2 (New York: Livingstone).

Kenny, A. (1992) *Aristotle on the Perfect Life* (Oxford: Oxford University Press).

MacIntyre, A. (1985) *After Virtue*, 2nd edn (London: Duckworth).

Oakley, A. (1985) *The Sociology of Housework* (New York: Basil Blackwell).

Witz, A. (1992) *Patriarchy and Professions* (London: Routledge).

Wright, C.J. and Hearn, J. (1993) The invisible man in nursing, Paper presented at the International Conference on Nursing, Women's History and the Politics of Welfare, University of Nottingham, 21–24 July.

CHAPTER THREE

Change and nursing

EDITOR'S INTRODUCTION

Traditional philosophical accounts of the phenomenon of change suppose that change must involve an object that persists through the change. Trevor Hussey argues that this view of change is highly questionable in its application to changes such as those in ideas or beliefs, those in values and those in theory. In these instances, there seems to be no underlying object of change. Trevor Hussey suggests that the kinds of change relevant to nursing are evolutionary changes, of which he identifies two kinds: Lamarckian and Darwinian. He claims that the former is the more relevant to the analysis of changes in theories, patterns of beliefs and so on.

Hussey draws attention to the fact that, in recent years, attempts have been made to characterise the nature of the changes that occur in scientific theorising. Typically, in science, theories are adopted and then jettisoned as they lose favour. Certain attempts to describe this pattern of change have recruited the language of theories of evolution. For example, theories may be said to 'compete' for acceptance. In this competition, the 'fitter' theories survive while weaker ones perish. As Trevor Hussey puts it, '[Scientific] theories are analogous to biological species; they compete with each other in a hostile environment of experimental text and critical evaluation, and the "fittest" theories survive while the rest are abandoned...' (see p. 56).

Trevor Hussey suggests that, if this model of change applies appropriately to scientific theories, it is plausible to suppose it to apply to nursing. It is well known that, at present, a variety of nursing models and theories are competing with each other for wide acceptance. As Hussey argues, the adoption of a Lamarckian model of evolutionary change leads to certain analyses of theory development in nursing which are potentially very fruitful indeed.

Change and nursing

Trevor Hussey

It seems hardly necessary to point out to nurses the significance and ubiquity of change: they have enjoyed or suffered an over-abundance of it in recent years. From the simplest of routine tasks to the most complex nursing procedures, from learning to use a new piece of equipment to the development of new nursing theories, and from the day-to-day arrangement of duty rosters to the very nature of the organisations in which they work, nurses have experienced a glut of fundamental changes.

Whether such changes are imposed upon the profession or are initiated by nurses themselves, the main concerns are practical: how to cope with the new ideas or procedures and how to manage them in order to ensure that they constitute an improvement rather than a deterioration or mere change for change's sake. Given the nature of a nurse's job and the rate of change with which she must cope, this practical focus is understandable, but there remains a need to step back from the ferment of the workplace and consider more general issues – in the way in which philosophers do. The more practical tasks of initiating, facilitating, monitoring, controlling and managing change may be helped by a better understanding of its fundamental nature and the processes that bring it about.

This chapter will begin with a philosophical analysis of change and offer a criterion stating what something must be to be a change of any kind. We will then examine some of the various forms that extended change can take, focusing on what is the most important of these for nurses: evolutionary change.

Next, it will be argued that, in understanding evolutionary change, we have to identify the kinds of process or mechanism that can bring it about and that there are, essentially, two kinds of process: direct and indirect (Lamarckian or Darwinian). The following section will discuss the way in which philosophers have tried to apply these models of evolutionary change in areas outside biology, their original home. It will examine some of the problems involved and show that the popular preference for the Darwinian

49

over the Lamarckian process is mistaken when we are considering change in such areas as knowledge, science and nursing.

Last, I will explore ways in which these ideas and distinctions can be applied to changes in nursing theory and practice, thus enabling us to gain a better understanding of them.

CHANGE AND EVOLUTION

In our everyday speech, we employ a rich variety of words to talk about changes, movements and developments, and we use them with ease and flexibility. All sorts of things are said to change: the weather turns cold, fruit ripens, conversations become heated, people grow older, opinions shift, fashions and tastes change, theories are gradually neglected and friendships blossom. We talk just as freely about changes that do not involve time, when for example, we say that air gets thinner with altitude or a wall changes in height along its length.

The task of discovering what all these disparate ideas of change have in common – what it is that constitutes change in general – is obviously a formidable one, and it is not surprising that philosophers have narrowed the field somewhat by focusing on changes to physical objects over time. In his seminal analysis, Aristotle was concerned with changes in what he called 'primary substances', by which he meant such material objects as a man, a horse or a statue. In *Physics* (Aristotle 1984, vol. 1, iv, 14, 222b30–1; v, 1, 224a34–224b5) he claimed that there were four things intrinsic to any change:

(1) An initial state or condition from which the change begins.
(2) A different state or condition to which the change proceeds.
(3) Something which 'underlies' the change; a persisting subject to which the change occurs (that is, a primary substance).
(4) Time, in which all change takes place.

Change has been the subject of philosophical debate ever since, but many modern philosophers would accept a similar analysis: change occurs when an object has (or lacks) a property or feature at one time and the same object lacks (or has) that property or feature at later time (see, for example, Newton-Smith, 1980; Lombard, 1986). Notice how this account retains the idea that a change involves something – the subject of the change – which persists and retains its identity throughout, while certain of its properties or features are lost or gained.

Centuries of argument have produced many objections to this kind of analysis of change, but it is not my purpose to discuss them here. I merely want to address a weakness already hinted at: the fact that the account assumes that change must involve a physical object altering over time. This means that when we talk, as talk we do, of changes to such things as theories, ideas, meanings, minds and practices, our criterion of change cannot be applied directly. Since we are concerned here with changes in the activities of nurses, their ideas and values, their knowledge, beliefs, theories and models – just as much as with changes in such physical things as the apparatus nurses use or the uniforms they wear – it then seems that we need a more general analysis for our purposes.

The traditional account of change also means that when we talk of spatial changes, such as a needle changing in diameter along its length, we must be using 'change' in a figurative, analogical or metaphorical way. Many influential philosophers, such as McTaggart (1927, section 316) and Geach (1972, p. 304), have considered this to be self-evidently correct. However, I believe that a completely general criterion of change should embrace changes in all dimensions, even though it so happens that only temporal changes are of significance in this discussion.

In developing a more general criterion of change, we can begin from the observation that our concept of 'change' is related to our concept of 'difference'. Everyday speech is not always consistent, but there is generally a distinction made between the two. All change involves difference but the reverse is not true. When a nurse progresses from a student to a Sister, she changes and becomes different in various respects, but an individual student is different from all other students without change being involved. As we have seen, Aristotle pointed out that change involves a persisting subject to which the change occurs while difference does not. He also argued in his *Metaphysics* (Aristotle 1984, vol. 2, 1069b6–7) that we can always distinguish between that which changes and that which differs. If the nurse has black hair as a student but grey hair when a Sister, the nurse's hair has changed while its colour is different.

A complete analysis of change would involve distinguishing between the various kinds of difference – only some of which are relevant to change – and carefully defining the notion of a dimension (Hussey, 1994). However, the following criterion of change will suffice for our purposes: there is a change if and only if there is a subject S which persists and retains its identity over time, from time1 to time2, and there is a difference which is exhibited by a property, state or part, properly predicated of S, from time1 to time2.

For example, an NHS institution consisting of a hospital and its staff will have changed if it persists and retains its identity over time while becoming a Trust. A difference between not being a Trust and being a Trust is involved in this case. However, it would be incorrect, according to this criterion, to say that a hospital building had become a Trust because Trust status cannot be properly predicated of (attributed to) a building.

Our criterion specifies what something must be to be a change of any kind. However, the changes that concern us most in nursing as well as everyday life are extended changes, involving a multitude of differences. Such changes may be revolutionary, cyclical, random, repetitive and so on, but perhaps the most common and important are evolutionary.

'Evolution' is not a precise term, but, in general, evolutionary changes can be identified either by their characteristic form or their mode of generation. In form, they are extended changes involving a fairly smooth or orderly emergence of novelty, any given part beginning from where the previous part finished, without discontinuities. The movements of a dance or the improvement of a nursing technique might be said to evolve in this sense. However, the word 'evolve' stems from the Latin 'evolvere' – to unroll – and thus refers to a mode of generation. Although in talking of evolutionary change, this specific reference to unrolling is often absent, there may be a generative mechanism implied – an opening out, unfolding or emerging of what is hidden or what potentially exists. The development of an embryo is an evolutionary change in this sense. In biology, 'evolution' is used, as a technical term, to refer to both the emergence of new species and the gradual development or adaptive change of organisms. While any idea of unrolling or unfolding is excluded, it remains that, as with all evolutionary change, it makes sense to ask what mechanism or process is responsible.

To summarise: being a species of change, evolution requires a subject that persists along a dimension while having properties, states or parts that differ. What makes the change evolutionary is its form or the way in which it is produced. It is a continuous change involving a fairly smooth or orderly appearance of new features in such a way as to demand an explanation in terms of a generative process or mechanism. Clearly, many of the changes nurses have to cope with are of this kind, be they changes in practice or in theory.

MODELS OF EVOLUTIONARY CHANGE

There are many mechanisms or processes that can generate evolutionary change, but I suggest that it is possible to distinguish two basic kinds. The first I shall call *direct*, the second *indirect*.

A *direct* mechanism acts directly on the properties, states or parts of the subject of the change to produce a pattern of differences that takes an evolutionary form. For example, a potter works directly on the contours of a piece of clay in order to shape it into a vase – and the final shape can be said to evolve from the original amorphous mass. Similarly, a zygote may divide to produce a population of cells that organise themselves into the form of an embryo according to the genetic instructions they contain. In this case, the subject of the change is the lineage of cells produced by mitosis, while the differences are the mitotic divisions, migration of cells, folding of tissues and so on.

An *indirect* mechanism involves selection. The persisting subject has properties, states or parts that exhibit random differences (or, at least, a pattern of differences unrelated to the subsequent evolution), and the mechanism involves a process of selection that eliminates some of these differences (or 'variations') in such a way that an evolutionary pattern of change results. A horticulturist might produce new varieties of rose in this way. The lineage of plants produced by seeds or cuttings would be the subject of the change, while the evolution would be brought about by the horticulturist selecting from the random variations shown by the plants in order slowly to bring about the rose he or she desires.

I suggest that all evolutionary changes are produced by either a direct or an indirect mechanism, or by both working together. A manager may employ a direct process to evolve a new bureaucratic regime in a hospital, deliberately introducing new procedures and systems according to a preconceived plan. However, he or she may also introduce a number of novel ideas before selecting those that appear to work and eliminating those that do not, thus employing an indirect process.

Theories of organic evolution provide important examples of both kinds of mechanism or process. The theory produced by Jean-Babtiste de Lamarck at the beginning of the 19th century is an important example of a direct mechanism, while the theory offered by Charles Darwin in the middle of the same century is a prime example of an indirect mechanism. It will be useful to give a brief description of both.

Lamarck gave several versions of his theory, none of which were very precise or clear (see Lamarck 1809; 1815–1822), but it appears to have two components, both of which are varieties of direct mechanism. The first claims that even the simplest of living organisms has a 'power of life' that drives it to develop, over many generations, towards ever greater complexity and 'perfection'. Thus, there is a chain of species from the lowest up to the highest, the latter being, at present, *Homo sapiens*. Species do not become extinct as they develop into the next because the lower end of the chain is constantly being replenished by a process of spontaneous generation of the simplest organisms from inorganic matter. This component of his theory is both factually incorrect – about spontaneous generation, for example – and useless as an explanation of evolution. It says merely that life evolves because it has the power to do so.

The second component of Lamarck's theory concerns the effect of the environment on living organisms. The conditions in which organisms live vary from place to place and time to time, and in doing so they alter the needs of the organisms. For example, arid conditions might harden the soil, making it more difficult for a mole to dig for the worms upon which it lives. The organism will then respond by modifying its behaviour and, if the need persists long enough, the new behaviour will become a habit – the mole will dig with increased effort and vigour. The habitual increase in use of the relevant organs or limbs will eventually lead to their enlargement – the mole will develop massive shoulder muscles and forelimbs. In this way the *individual organism* will become adapted to its changed environment. Lamarck believed that the species to which the organism belongs will then be transformed because the enlarged organs and limbs of each individual will be passed on to the next generation – thus the baby moles will inherit their parents' muscles.

There are two well-known criticisms of this second component of Lamarck's theory of evolution. First, it is claimed, perhaps unjustly, that the theory explains evolution in terms of wants and conscious strivings on the part of the organisms. Second, it assumes, wrongly, that features acquired during the lifetime of an individual organism can be passed on to its offspring. Modern science tells us that only changes in the germplasm of an organism's gonads can be transmitted.

However, there is a more fundamental criticism to be made: Lamarck's theory is unacceptable not because it gives a false explanation of organic evolution but because it offers no explanation at all. It *assumes* that an organism will respond to a need by altering its behaviour, that this will develop into a habit, that the increased use of certain organs will cause them to grow larger and stronger, but it does not explain why these things would occur. A mole could respond to hard soil by crying itself to sleep; its muscles, if exercised, could remain unchanged or merely turn green. Lamarck explains neither the nature of the causal mechanisms involved nor why they are in place. In contrast, it is generally accepted that Darwin's theory can explain such things.

However, it is important to notice what these criticisms of Lamarck's theory do and do not establish. They show that his theory is unacceptable as an explanation of organic evolution as it occurs on Earth. This is because it assumes the existence of causal processes that either do not exist – as in the case of the 'inheritance of acquired characters' – or which exist for reasons unexplained by the theory. This does not, however, mean that a similar theory could not be perfectly satisfactory in such other areas as the evolution of science, culture or nursing, as will be seen below.

Modern biologists accept that organic evolution is produced by an indirect process, essentially as described by Darwin (1859) but modified to embrace our better understanding of genetics. Darwin proposed that evolution is produced by a process of natural selection acting on 'blind' variations. In a population of organisms, even of a single species, the individuals will differ, in varying degrees, from each other. If the organisms are competing with each other for limited resources, and struggling to exist in a hostile environment, some of the variations will be advantageous and some disadvantageous to the individuals possessing them. Thus, in a given environment, those individuals possessing certain characteristics will have a greater chance of surviving and reproducing than will those that do not possess them. If the characteristics are genetically determined (that is, heritable) then, in the next generation, an increased proportion of the organisms will possess the advantageous characteristics, and so on over many generations, producing evolutionary change. The differences or variations are 'blind' in the sense that the form they take and the time at which they occur are unconnected with the demands placed upon the organisms by natural selection: genetic mutations occur by chance.

Amongst the benighted moles, some will have slightly larger muscles and stronger limbs, some will respond to hunger by digging harder and some will possess physiologies that ensure that, when they exercise, their muscles will respond by enlarging. Such individuals will be more likely to survive than those lacking these features, and, as long as the features are heritable, they will be more common in the next generation of moles.

Although Darwin was concerned with describing the mechanism at work in the biological world, his theory can be generalised to apply in other areas. As we shall see, many philosophers have claimed that it is an essentially Darwinian process that has brought about the evolution of knowledge, the development of science, cultural changes and so on.

APPLYING THE MODELS: EVOLUTIONARY EPISTEMOLOGY

Over the past 25 years or so, many philosophers have become interested in borrowing ideas from evolutionary biology and applying them to areas such as the growth of knowledge and the development of science. This 'evolutionary epistemology' has given rise to two programmes of investigation (Bradie, 1986). One concerns itself with the evolution of our cognitive mechanisms and capacities, and the implications this evolution has for explaining the ways in which we perceive and understand the world. This is, arguably (Plotkin, 1994), as much a scientific enterprise as a philosophical one and is not our primary concern.

The programme of interest here stems from the work of Toulmin (1972), Popper (1974, 1975, 1979, 1984) and Campbell (1977), and uses theories and ideas from evolutionary biology to illuminate the way in which concepts, beliefs, knowledge and (especially) scientific theories evolve over time. Philosophers have produced several different accounts, and the debate continues (see, for example, Ruse, 1986; Radnitzky and Bartley, 1987; Richards, 1987; Hull, 1988), but the basic idea is that a Darwinian process is at work. Such things as scientific theories are analogous to biological species: they compete with each other in a hostile environment of experimental test and critical evaluation, and the 'fittest' theories survive while the rest are abandoned. Of course, scientists can improve the prospects of their favoured theory, in this struggle for existence, by introducing novel variations in the form of additions or amendments. In this way, an individual theory can evolve.

Apart from clarifying the way in which knowledge or science has developed, evolutionary epistemologists also hope to explain such things as the progress and rationality of science. It is widely believed that science accumulates knowledge and gives us theories of ever-increasing accuracy and predictive power. Unlike, for example, fashions in clothes, science does not merely change: it makes progress. The Darwinian process of selection, it is said, ensures that the *better* theories survive. We may not be able to claim that our latest scientific theories are wholly true – after all, they have often proved false in the past – but we can at least be sure that they are an improvement on what has gone before.

Similarly, during the past 350 years, science has come to be seen as a paradigm of rationality. It can give rational justifications of its knowledge claims and theories. Indeed, the opinions of scientists are invoked to settle disputes about everything from mad cow disease to juvenile delinquency, in much the same way that theologians would have been consulted in medieval times. Unfortunately, it has proved very difficult to explain exactly how the scientific method works and why it justifies our faith in its products. Thus, it is tempting to suggest that science is rational not because of the methods used by individual scientists but because the whole scientific enterprise consists of systematically subjecting its theories to the rigours of a Darwinian process of selection.

The focus here is on science because that has been the subject of the debate in evolutionary epistemology, but we are primarily concerned with nursing. Although science and nursing are very different activities, both can be seen as social practices that employ theories and develop a body of knowledge and skills, and both evolve over time. Hence, we can speculate how this brand of evolutionary epistemology might be applied in nursing; this will be the subject of the next section.

Before embarking on that project, we need to make sure that we have properly identified the processes involved. For, despite the widespread agreement that the Darwinian model is the appropriate one, there are good reasons for thinking otherwise. These will be stated briefly as there is not enough space to present the arguments in detail.

We can start by noticing that the pattern and speed of change in science contrast markedly with those seen in biological evolution. The latter is generally depicted as a tree that branches repeatedly, so that it would multiply species indefinitely were it not for the termination of some of the branches by extinction. Science – at least natural science – is, however, claimed to progress by producing theories of ever-increasing generality, which subsume their predecessors, thus turning the biological pattern upside down (Popper, 1979; Ruse, 1986). As to the rate of change, although it is not a simple matter to make comparisons, it is intuitively obvious that change in social practices such as science is much more rapid than organic evolution. These are not, however, conclusive arguments because a Darwinian process may produce different effects in dissimilar situations.

A much more serious objection to the Darwinian account of evolutionary epistemology concerns the origin of innovations: the variations or differences necessary for change. It is an essential

feature of the indirect model offered by Darwin that the variations
are 'blind', in the sense that their timing, and the form they take, is
unconnected to the selection pressures or 'demands of the environment' faced by the organisms. However, it can be argued that, in
science, innovations are devised deliberately and purposefully: modifications to theories, new hypotheses, redesigned apparatus, novel
procedures and so on are introduced precisely to overcome the difficulties encountered. Many philosophers have recognised this objection (see the summary in Bradie, 1986), although they cling to the
Darwinian model in evolutionary epistemology despite this. It should
be noticed, however, that the process at work in science is exactly in
accord with a direct or Lamarckian model of evolutionary change, in
which the demands of the environment act on whatever is evolving
in order to induce appropriate changes.

Similarly, in the Darwinian model, natural selection is as blind as
the variations upon which it works: there is no direction or purpose.
Several commentators (for example, Hull, 1982; Bechtel, 1984;
Richards, 1987) have pointed out that this is not the case in the
evolution of science, in which at least part of the selective process
involves human decision and choice. The survival of a theory or the
abandonment of a programme of research depends not only on the
empirical 'facts', but also on prevailing scientific paradigms, intellectual fashions, economic resources, political prejudices and so on.
Such factors are clearly even more prevalent in the case of nursing
where, for example, financial cut-backs can eliminate worthy activities while leaving less useful, but more powerful, ones entrenched.
Again, this account of the action of the environment fits the Lamarckian model, in which the subject of the evolution is induced to
change in a specific direction.

Finally, the transmission of innovations in science is very un-
Darwinian. In the organic world, information is transmitted down the
generations by genetic inheritance, which has important implications
for the evolutionary process. However advantageous it may be, a new
mutation will take many generations to spread through the population as natural selection gets to work. In science, new ideas and practices spread rapidly amongst the scientific community in a manner
analogous to the Lamarckian process of the inheritance of acquired
characters. Furthermore, in science, ideas and practices can be resurrected from long-abandoned theories and borrowed from other disciplines, but in the organic world, when a species becomes extinct, its
genetic material dies with it and, except for the relatively rare
phenomena of hybridisation and 'genetic engineering', genetic mate-

rial from one species cannot be transferred to another, however useful it might be.

In borrowing concepts from biology, evolutionary epistemologists have generally assumed that the subject of change – that which persists and retains its identity throughout – will be analogous to a species. Unfortunately, this ignores the vigorous debate within the philosophy of biology concerning the nature of species and their function in evolution (Ereshefsky, 1992). For reasons beyond the scope of this paper, it will be accepted here that the subject of evolutionary change is best seen as a *lineage* – a series of entities produced by a generative relation such as the ancestor–descendant relationship that operates between the generations of a family (Hussey, 1994). It is the lineage that can be said to evolve, while the individual entities making up the lineage are the products of that evolution.

In summary, although there is no doubt that the process at work in biological evolution is an indirect or Darwinian one, when we turn our attention to the evolution of social practices, such as science and nursing, we see that a direct model – akin to the second component of Lamarck's theory – is more apposite. The usual objections to his ideas no longer bite: the conscious strivings of scientists are a part of the evolutionary mechanism, and the transmission of the novel variations is closely analogous to the inheritance of acquired characters. It remains true that his theory does not explain why these processes are in place, but, although we need a Darwinian explanation for the existence of the psychological capacities that make science possible, this does not mean that these capacities must also work in a Darwinian way or that their products must evolve by this kind of process.

What of the progress and rationality of science and, we hope, of such activities as nursing? There are bonuses here for adopting a Lamarckian model. Progress involves the notion of change for the better: it is an evaluative concept. The Darwinian theory cannot explain the success of science because it is a theory of change rather than of progress. Selection is not goal-directed: it merely ensures that organisms fit prevailing conditions. Adopting the Darwinian theory removed the locus of rationality from the individual scientists to the process in general, but the Lamarckian model returns it to the intellectual and skilled activities of the people involved. Science makes progress because it achieves goals we value by means of the creativity, skills and understanding of those who work in it, and it is reasonable to suggest that the same is true of nursing.

CHANGE IN NURSING

It is obvious that nursing develops and that many of the changes have the evolutionary form described earlier. Whether it makes progress is, perhaps, a little more contentious, but only the most cynical would deny that, over the long term, some things improve, while allowing that some do not. If we can understand these changes, we will be able to see why they take the form they do and how we might influence the process in order to achieve the changes we want. Gaining this understanding requires a detailed study of the various elements and processes involved. This is not, itself, a philosophical task, but if we are to understand change properly and learn how to handle it better in the future, we need to find the most accurate and useful ways of conceptualising and describing the processes involved so that we can identify the vital components: this is where the philosopher can make a contribution.

If the analysis presented above is correct, we need to start with the general criterion of change offered above, and identify the various persisting subjects of change and their properties, states or parts that can exhibit differences of the relevant kinds; here, the dimension of change is obviously time. Many of the most important of these changes will take an evolutionary form, and it has been argued that, if we want to understand how these are generated, we will do well to adopt a direct or Lamarckian model. If this is so, we must try to identify the various forces in the 'environment' in which nursing takes place that may be responsible for inducing changes. Where human agents are involved, we need to identify the theories, values, principles and prejudices that make them modify nursing practices in the way they do. Similarly, we need to note those elements in nursing practice and education that respond to the demands placed upon them by the 'environment' in order to generate the changes. This chapter will end with a brief elaboration of these points.

Nursing is a complex and dynamic collection of social practices. It involves a host of practical and intellectual activities in constant interaction with each other and with a wider environment consisting of institutions, other professional groups, patients, their families and the wider social setting, right up (or down) to the prevailing political and economic systems. Change is generated within nursing as a result of these interactions.

As it changes, nursing is best seen as a skein of threads, each thread a bundle of evolving lineages, each lineage a succession of entities slightly modified from its predecessor. One substantial thread will consist of lineages of nursing practices, another of theories, another of training courses, another of career structures and so on. From modes of dress to codes of conduct, wherever developments have occurred it should be possible to identify evolving lineages, some coming into being and others terminating.

For example, those involved in nurse education will know that there has been a bewildering proliferation of nursing theories and models. Some are modifications of earlier theories; some are original enough to constitute the beginning of a new lineage. Some rapidly disappear, but those that attract the attention of nurses, nurse educators and theorists will begin to change. Modified versions will appear in response to criticisms or a changing focus of interest, and in this way a new lineage of theories will evolve. Some innovations – the idea of holism, for example – will prove so popular that they will spread rapidly; other lineages will 'acquire that character'.

A full understanding of the changes would include identifying the components of the Lamarckian process involved: the mechanisms by which new theories are generated, what factors in the nursing environment stimulate the innovations, and what reasoning, sentiment or ideological commitments colour the responses. To evaluate the changes and decide whether they constitute progress is another matter. It involves asking the purpose and value of nursing theories and models, and discovering what critical forces need to be developed within the nursing community to enable it to induce 'improving' and useful innovations or weed out worthless or incoherent theories.

By far the thickest thread in the evolving skein of nursing consists of the countless practical tasks that occupy the working day. Receiving new patients on the ward, changing dressings, dealing with paperwork, calming fears and distributing drugs – the list is endless. However, each of these practices develops over time in response to new knowledge, technical innovations, changing budgets and so on. They, too, form lineages that evolve for the better or worse, and they need to be understood and evaluated.

To help us depict this process, we might borrow some distinctions from action theory. Actions are specific intentional pieces of behaviour performed by human agents, for example raising an arm, grasping and walking. Acts are socially defined happenings involving actions, which have a meaning within a community and which take place in socially defined situations. They are goal-directed in that they are defined in terms of what is achieved if they are successful; in this, they are normative, since our performance of them can succeed or fail. Acts vary from such simple things as greetings, farewells and insults to such complex things as playing a game or marrying; and complex acts may have lesser acts within them. They may involve various 'props', for example, instruments, tools or furniture. The nursing community shares the repertoire available in the wider community but has acts of its own such as taking a temperature, 'handing over' between shifts and writing a care plan. The performance of an act involves rule-governed sequences of actions, the rules being determined by the community and subject to change. Some of the actions constituting an act are essential, others are arbitrary, but it is not a simple matter to tell which is which, and this makes rational change difficult. A child growing up in a community or a student nurse entering her profession must learn the repertoire of acts available and the rules for performing them correctly.

These distinctions enable us to identify the components in the evolutionary process. Each performance of an act is a part of a lineage of similar acts, and the generative mechanism is the process of teaching and learning within nursing. As innovations occur – as new apparatus is adopted or the rules for performing the act are modified – so the lineage will evolve. For example, the act of 'taking a temperature' has evolved by the replacement of mercury glass thermometers, perhaps first by disposable chemical dot devices and then by tympanic thermometers. This has been accompanied by changes in the activities of the nurse, not least a reduction in the time taken, from several minutes to a few seconds. Here, it was largely pressure for efficiency and safety that produced the innovations, but questions of convenience, reliability and cost may also have decided the kinds of device used.

Of course, not all change involves technological developments in this way. For example, the attitude towards allowing parents to visit on children's wards has been transformed in recent decades. Parents can now stay overnight, help care for their child and even accompany their children to the anaesthetic room in surgical cases. These changes have been brought about gradually by pressure from parents and progressive nurses, backed by research and government committee reports, while the developments have also been modified by staffing levels, the attitudes of managers and other environmental forces. Clearly, however, considerations of efficiency and cost-effectiveness should have less influence here. Indeed, sometimes purely symbolic or ritualistic factors are most important – as when bereaved relatives are offered tea in china cups rather than plastic beakers, ejected with whatever cost-effectiveness from a machine.

Such changes as these, and the innovations they involve, may seem simple in retrospect. Similarly, with the benefit of hindsight we can see which changes have been retrogressive and which progressive. We are apt to wonder why those involved – presumably just as clever as we are – took so long and made so many mistakes. However, past changes are easy; it is the future ones that are more difficult. One way to help to ensure that nursing evolves as we feel it should is to understand the processes at work, to clarify the concepts we employ in thinking about its development and to equip ourselves with a realistic theory of change. This is intended to be a contribution to that task.

ACKNOWLEDGEMENT

I would like to thank Claire Hussey, RGN, RSCN, for her help with this article.

REFERENCES

Aristotle (1984) *The Complete Works of Aristotle: The Revised Oxford Translation,* vols. 1 and 2, Barnes, J. (ed.) (Princeton: Princeton University Press).

Bechtel, W. (1984) The evolution of our understanding of the cell: a study in the dynamics of scientific progress, *Studies in History and Philosophy of Science,* **15**: 309–56.

Bradie, M. (1986) Assessing evolutionary epistemology, *Biology and Philosophy,* **1**: 401–59.

Campbell, D.T. (1974) Evolutionary epistemology, in Schilpp, P.A. (ed.) *The Philosophy of Karl Popper,* pp. 413–63 (La Salle: Open Court).

Campbell, D.T. (1977) Comments on the 'natural selection model of conceptual evolution', *Philosophy of Science,* **44**: 502–7.

Darwin, C. (1859) *The Origin of Species.* Reprinted 1968 (London: John Murray) (Harmondsworth: Penguin).

Ereshefsky, M. (ed.) (1992) *The Units of Evolution: Essays on the Nature of Species* (Cambridge, MA: MIT Press).

Geach, P.T. (1972) *Logic Matters* (Oxford: Basil Blackwell).

Hull, D. (1982) The naked meme, in Plotkin, H.C. (ed.) *Learning, Development and Culture,* pp. 273–327 (Chichester: John Wiley).

Hull, D. (1988) *Science as a Process: An Evolutionary Account of the Social and Conceptual Development of Science* (Chicago: University of Chicago Press).

Hussey, T.B. (1994) Some philosophical aspects of change and evolution, Unpublished doctoral thesis, Bodleian Library, Oxford.

Lamarck, J-B (1809) *Philosophie Zoologique, ou Exposition des Considérations Relatives a l'Histoire Naturelle des Animaux,* 2 vols. Trans. Elliot, H. *Zoological Philosophy* (1914) (London: Macmillan).

Lamarck, J-B (1815–1822) *Histoire Naturelle des Animaux sans Vertèbres,* 7 vols. [Natural History of Invertebrates] (Paris).

Lombard, L.B. (1986) *Events: A Metaphysical Study* (London: Routledge & Kegan Paul).

McTaggart, J.M.E. (1927) *The Nature of Existence* (Cambridge: Cambridge University Press).

Newton-Smith, W.H. (1980) *The Structure of Time* (London: Routledge & Kegan Paul).

Plotkin, H.C. (1987) Evolutionary epistemology as science, *Biology and Philosophy,* **2**: 295–313.

Plotkin, H.C. (1991) The testing of evolutionary epistemology, *Biology and Philosophy,* **6**: 481–97.

Plotkin, H.C. (1994) *Darwin Machines and the Nature of Knowledge* (Harmondsworth: Penguin).

Popper, K.R. (1974) Darwinism as a metaphysical research programme, in Schilpp, P.A. (ed.) *The Philosophy of Karl Popper,* pp. 133–43 (La Salle: Open Court).

Popper, K.R. (1975) The rationality of scientific revolutions, (Herbert Spencer Lectures 1973), in Hacking, I. (ed.) (1981) *Scientific Revolutions,* pp. 80–106 (Oxford: Oxford University Press).

Popper, K.R. (1979) *Objective Knowledge* (rev. edn) (Oxford: Clarendon Press).

Popper, K.R. (1984) Evolutionary epistemology, in Pollard, J.W. (ed.) *Evolutionary Theory: Paths into the Future,* pp. 239–55 (London: John Wiley).

Radnitzky, G. and Bartley, W.W. (eds) (1987) *Evolutionary Epistemology, Rationality and the Sociology of Knowledge* (La Salle: Open Court).

Richards, R.J. (1987) *Darwin and the Emergence of Evolutionary Theories of Mind and Behaviour* (Chicago: University of Chicago Press).

Ruse, M. (1986) *Taking Darwin Seriously* (Oxford: Blackwell).

Toulmin, S. (1972) *Human Understanding* (Oxford: Oxford University Press).

Part II

CONCEPTUAL FOUNDATIONS

CHAPTER FOUR

Holism in nursing

EDITOR'S INTRODUCTION

The concept of holism is widely appealed to in nursing literature. Furthermore, it seems universally paraded as a 'good thing'. To describe a regime of care as holistic is to expect its instant approval.

As much as holism is lauded in nursing, its opposite – reductionism – is deplored. A regime of care that claimed to be reductionist could safely anticipate widespread scorn, but the stampede away from reductionism in order to embrace holism is deeply problematic. Simon Woods points out that it is far from obvious that holism has a straightforward application to nursing. For example, does holism exclude specialisation? What are the 'wholes' that holism includes – people, families, cultures...? Any attempt to answer these questions needs to specify just what it is that is embraced when one adopts holism. It is then necessary to see how holism, once defined, might apply to the nursing context and whether its application is warranted.

Simon Woods' chapter provides a clear path through these important problems. He clarifies the ideas central to holism and shows how they apply in nursing practice. He goes on to identify Strong and Weak versions of holism. The Strong version is shown to be highly problematic, but the Weak version is endorsed.

Holism in nursing

Simon Woods

There is a puzzle at the centre of nursing that concerns the understanding and value of holism. Nursing itself is often characterised as holistic (Jacono and Jacono, 1994); at other times, it is patients who are described as holistic (Rogers, 1970, 1980); at other times still, it is the responses of patients to nursing care that are described as holistic (Kolcaba, 1992, 1994).

Owen and Holmes (1993, p. 1688) refer to holism as 'a turbid, amorphic term, of Quixotic character, the meaning of which alters according to the context in which it is located'. Nevertheless, holism is a concept deemed to be highly significant for nursing, hence its prevalence throughout the literature. To use this concept effectively, it is important to try and be precise about its meaning (Allen, 1991). This chapter will attempt to clarify the meaning of holism and, in doing so, unravel part of the puzzle already introduced. It should be noted, as Owen and Holmes (1993, p. 1688) remind us, that 'holism is not a single unitary concept and we ought rather to speak of "holisms"'. With this comment in mind, it is still possible to identify a number of specific applications of holism to nursing.

A simple definition of holism is that: things are more than simply the sum of their constituent parts (cf. Smuts, 1926; Owen and Holmes, 1993). Therefore, things described as holistic share the common property that any reduction to their constituent parts is not sufficient to account for the whole; something of defining importance is lost in such an analysis.

With regard to the question of what the value of holism is to nursing, there are several problem areas in the claim that nursing is holistic. This chapter will deal with two of these. One such difficulty is that nursing is becoming increasingly specialised (Cribb et al., 1994). Specialism itself can be seen to focus on particular parts or features, be these diseases, therapies or practices. The second problem concerns the appropriate methodology for nursing research.

This chapter will also consider some of the historical influences on the development of the concept of holism. It will be shown that there are two definitions or theories of holism operating within nursing. It will be argued that one of these theories is too strong and entails too many contradictions with nursing practice. The second, and arguably preferable, theory is weaker and more compatible with the wide spectrum of nursing practice.

The reasons for developing this debate here are two-fold: first, to introduce some of the background issues associated with the complex concept of holism, and second, to introduce the application of philosophical analysis to nursing theory.

WHAT IS HOLISM?

This question will be approached from two directions: first, from a philosophical perspective, and second, from a more applied nursing perspective. This will provide an opportunity to introduce some relevant terminology and to illustrate the connection between these two approaches.

Earlier, a definition of holism was proffered: things are more than simply the sum of their constituent parts. One way of exploring this statement is through a 'thought experiment'. This is a technique often used by philosophers to test out certain theories, rather like the way in which a manufacturer will test out a new car. In the safety of the mental laboratory, the theory can be put through its paces, its performance can be tested to the limits and its weaknesses identified.

The concept of holism seems to capture an important feature of objects, processes and events. Take, for example, the property of 'softness'. Imagine that you have a favourite pillow that is your favourite because of the fact that it is so soft. The softness is an important, if not essential, element of the pillow, but how can the property of 'softness' be explained? One solution may involve a close examination of the pillow. In this way, various measurements of size and weight could be taken. The material of which the pillow is made could be examined under a microscope and the composition and organisation of the component fibres noted. An exhaustive list of the parts and dimensions could then be compiled. But where on that list would the softness be? The softness of the pillow, it seems, is not another part of the pillow such as the fabric or the colour, yet it is a property of the pillow since it is this specific property that makes the pillow your favourite. Adding together the constituent parts of the pillow does not constitute an adequate account of what the pillow is to you. It seems that the sum or total of those parts is formed in such a way that other, equally defining, properties emerge. The particular softness of the pillow, which is so pleasing to you, is an 'emergent' property that is not captured by the list of component parts, no matter how extensive. The pillow needs to be seen as a whole and also seen within the context of its use, for this important property to be realised.

The failure to capture all of the properties of the pillow by an analysis of its component parts is an argument for the importance of holism. Holism, as illustrated by this example, is often contrasted with analysis as a means of capturing the complex range of properties that an object, event or process may exhibit. The process of analysis is often described as 'reductionist' because it reduces a complex thing to its most simple parts.

The holism of nursing is frequently contrasted with 'reductionism' in nursing literature (Liaschenko and Davis, 1991). For example, nursing is often described as 'holistic', in contrast to some aspects of medicine, which are described as 'reductionist'. One way of defining a concept such as holism is by negative definition, by contrasting the term with a range of opposites. Holism is often negatively defined by contrast with reductionism and other concepts such as 'scientific', 'quantification' and 'positivism' (Holmes, 1990). This is strongly expressed by Griffin (1993, p. 310), who writes, 'Holism is against all forms of reductionism.'

If holism is a useful concept in nursing, a more positive definition is required: for a concept such as holism to be useful, it needs to be employed with some degree of precision. The soft pillow example is a simplification of the issues relevant to this discussion. In particular, the example does not deal with a whole range of complex philosophical questions and objections, but it is advantageous in that it provides a starting point.

What is clear from the example is that there are two central issues that need to be explored if the connection between holism and nursing is to be discussed. The first issue concerns knowledge and how it is gained. This issue was implicit in the above example, since one kind of explanation of the softness of the pillow is to say how we 'know' that the pillow is soft. Questions about the nature of knowledge and how knowledge is gained come under the technical philosophical term 'epistemology'.

The second and related issue concerns the way in which the kinds of things that exist are described. This comes under the technical philosophical description of 'metaphysics'. Nursing theory makes implicit and explicit reference to epistemology and metaphysics (Rogers, 1970; Sarter, 1988). All people hold metaphysical beliefs even though they may never reflect upon them. Take, for example, the simple fact of stepping out of bed in the morning. Most people do not initially stretch out a tentative toe to test whether the floor of the bedroom is still there! We expect the floor to be there owing to a set of beliefs we have about physical objects, for example, that physical objects exist and that they exist over time unless caused not to do so. So, in the absence of an earthquake, fire or explosion, we awake with the certainty that the floor of the bedroom will still be where we left it the night before. Hence, it is reasonable to assume that most people have metaphysical beliefs including beliefs about physical objects. A moment's reflection will show that most people have a metaphysical description of the world that is quite comprehensive.

The connection between epistemology and metaphysics can be explained by further developing the pillow example. This began with the question of how to account for the softness of a favourite pillow. One approach to answering the question is to assume that, by breaking down or analysing the pillow into its constituent parts, the 'softness' could be identified as a constituent part or else analysed out. Since no constituent part corresponding to the softness of the pillow has been identified, it could be argued that the property of softness is explained away by the process of analysis, so that what is 'really' there is the sum of the constituent parts of the pillow.

This argument assumes both an epistemology and a metaphysics. The metaphysics, that is, the description of what there is, assumes that a very complex world can be adequately described by reducing it to its constituent parts, so that what exists can be exhaustively described by a list of these constituents. The softness of the pillow can be accounted for in terms of the combination of the constituents of the pillow.

The epistemological assumptions of this account are that knowledge of the way the world really is can be gained through a process of analysis or reduction to more fundamental quantifiable constituents. These provide the foundations upon which knowledge is built. This account was described above as reductionism, and, although the term is a neutral adjective, reductionism has come to be regarded as pejorative by many nurse commentators (Holmes, 1990; Webb, 1993). because reductionism seems to omit aspects of the world that are important to people in general and to nursing in particular.

It is important to recognise that the holism/reductionism debate and the criticisms levelled at reductionism are not unique to nursing scholarship. This debate in nursing theory reflects a wider historical debate, which derives from the development of modern scientific thinking in the 17th century. The emergence of modern science is associated with such concepts as reductionism and quantification (Harre, 1989). Over the past three centuries, science has demonstrated increasing explanatory and predictive powers. Because science has been successful, it has proved a powerful force and an influential conceptual model. This issue will be explored further below.

From the simple pillow example, a competing anti-reductionist epistemology and metaphysics can be developed. In this competing view, the softness of the pillow is seen as an important, if not essential, property of the pillow in question. This particular property of the pillow, far from being explained away by the reductionist analysis described above, is in fact completely ignored. The consequence of ignoring this property fails to capture a distinct feature of the world and fails to capture the importance or value of the pillow in respect of this property.

The metaphysical assumptions of the anti-reductionist or holistic argument are that the world contains not only constituent parts, but also properties and values that cannot be explained in terms of the constituent parts. The epistemological assumptions of this holistic argument are that knowledge of the world requires questions not only about constituent parts, but also about the properties of parts when they are combined as wholes. This alternative anti-reductionist/holist account should be seen as analogous to the wider historical debate introduced above and to the more familiar debate chronicled in the nursing literature (Holmes, 1990).

An example closer to home may make the point more clearly. Despite any beneficial value the experience of pain may have, for example, as a warning of damage, pain is generally regarded as an unpleasant experience. It is usually considered by nurses as a phenomenon to be noted and relieved. Utilising the contrasting approaches outlined above, the value of holism can be explored by considering the following case.

Case example

Bob is a 45-year-old father of two teenage sons. He has carcinoma of the bronchus, which has metastasised to multiple sites in his skeleton. He has been admitted to hospital for pain relief and is taking 30 mg slow release morphine every 12 hours. Emma, Bob's wife, is seen to be tearful at visiting times, and Bob is observed to be very short-tempered with his sons.

Approach 1 (reductionist)

This patient has metastatic bone cancer. One effect of this disease process is the release of prostaglandins, chemicals known to act as irritants to terminal peripheral nerve endings. The effect of this interaction is a powerful afferent neurotransmission to the brain, resulting in a localised pain sensation that is indicated by such behaviour as guarding and immobilisation of the affected part. As the noxious stimulation becomes cognisable by the cerebral cortex, verbal behaviours such as involuntary noises are observed and descriptions such as 'aching' and 'throbbing' used by the subject.

Psychological behaviours such as depression or irritability may be observed. A group of compounds known collectively as non-steroidal anti-inflammatory drugs (NSAIDs) are known to exert a powerful inhibiting effect on prostaglandins. An example from this group of compounds is prescribed for Bob and he is subsequently observed for pain behaviour and asked to use verbal descriptors to characterise his pain experience. No guarding is observed, Bob is more mobile and he says that he no longer experiences throbbing or aching.

Approach 2 (holistic)

Bob seems to be quiet and withdrawn. He does not talk to other patients in his bay and spends most of the day lying on his bed. The nurse goes over to Bob, sits down at the side of the bed, catches his eye and says, 'I hope I am not disturbing you. I thought that I would come over and see how things are.'

'I am fine,' Bob replies, looking down.

'It's just that you seem a little withdrawn.'

'I would be fine if people would just leave me alone, if I could just get comfortable.'

'Get comfortable?'

'Yes, my bones seem to ache and throb; I can't seem to get away from it and the pain killers don't touch it.'

'It sounds like we need to get on top of this pain straight away. Shall I bring you something stronger for the pain now?' Bob nods assent. 'When you are feeling better we can sit down together and you can tell me about your pain, where it is, what makes it better or worse and describe it in your own words – that way we can work together to find the best way of managing your pain. Is that OK?'

'Yes but, I don't want to be doped up, I don't want to be sleeping all the time; I see little enough of the family as it is!'

'I can understand how important that must be, but not all pain medicines make you drowsy and there are other things, things you can do to help yourself which can help; sometimes it's helpful just to talk.'

'Yes, OK, I will give it a try, I may feel more like talking if I could get rid of this aching.'

'OK Bob, I will just go and get that medication for you.'

The nurse goes away to discuss with the doctor the prescription of an NSAID. She makes a mental note to try to catch Emma next time she visits, just to ask how she is coping.

Approaches 1 and 2 are fictional accounts designed to illustrate some of the points introduced in the pillow example. Approach 1 locates Bob's pain at the biochemical level; the language itself is reductionist because it reduces Bob's pain to a description of the constituents of the phenomenon, using objective, scientific language. The mechanics of the disease, the pain experience and the proposed treatment are all described in the same kind of language.

The implication of this approach is that Bob just happens to be an example of this phenomenon, the phenomenon will respond to the correct pharmacy and that this will be true for other examples of this kind.

Approach 2 places Bob himself as the focus of attention, recognising the context in which Bob is situated. The nurse relates to Bob as a person, first enquiring about his feelings and allowing him to identify what issues are salient for him. The nurse recognises that the pain requires treatment with appropriate medication and also that Bob's experience of pain is interwoven with other relevant aspects of his situation. For example, the nurse sees the possibility that Bob's pain may be having tangible effects on the rest of his family.

The language of Approach 2 centres on the interaction between Bob and the nurse and on the conversation. The nurse's use of communication skills reflects the nurse's insight into Bob's situation. It could be argued that Approach 2 is an holistic approach, in contrast to the reductionist account of Approach 1.

An important point could be advanced to the effect that, while Approach 1 is implicit within Approach 2, the reverse is not the case. This latter point requires further consideration (see below).

In this section, an attempt has been made to define holism; this has been achieved by contrasting holism with reductionism. A number of simple examples have been used to introduce some of the philosophical assumptions that underpin holism and its application to nursing. It has been suggested that the holism/reductionism debate has a wider historical context and that nursing theory has drawn heavily upon this background.

INFLUENCE OF HOLISM ON NURSING THOUGHT

In seeking a place for nursing as a discipline with a theoretical basis, a number of identifiable themes have been drawn on by scholars of nursing and the debate between holism and reductionism has its antecedents in the history of ideas.

A pivotal historical period is the 17th century, which marks the advent of modern thinking in philosophy and science. It is convenient to identify a particular figure, Rene Descartes (1596–1650), whose ideas have been influential in the framework of the contemporary debate. Cartesianism is the term given to theories influenced by Descartes.

Descartes' thinking covered both epistemology and metaphysics. Simply put, Descartes argued that the world consists of two, and only two, kinds of substance: mental substance and physical substance. Descartes came to this conclusion through a process of introspection, a series of what he termed 'meditations' (Descartes, 1977). Physical substances are characterised by their extension and their measurable, quantifiable properties. Mental substances are non-extended, characterised by psychological properties such as thinking and feeling. Descartes' account suggests that a person is a combination of both kinds of substance whereas a block of stone is a physical substance alone.

For Descartes and for some of those subsequently influenced by Cartesianism, physical substances could be further explored by combining observation with mathematics to create a method of investigating the physical world, of describing the physical world and, ultimately, of predicting the behaviour of things within the physical world.

These 'methods' have been influential on all aspects of modern life and many everyday nursing activities. Recording a person's temperature with a thermometer and plotting this on a graph is a more accurate way of recording a fever, and therefore possible response to treatment, than merely noting that the person is 'hot'.

From the 17th century, the development of the physical sciences accelerated and methods of science were refined. Science became predominantly interested in the quantification of physical substance to the exclusion of mental substance since, by definition, mental substances cannot be quantified because they are not extended. This resulted in a degree of scepticism over the existence of a mental substance at all. For some thinkers, this led to the assertion that only physical substance exists (physicalism), thus denying the other half of Cartesian dualism, namely the existence of mental substance.

The methods employed by the physical sciences have been effective as tools for investigation and prediction, thus providing a powerful model for other sciences. It is often argued that medicine has been influenced by this model since medicine uses many facts derived from the physical sciences, such as physics and chemistry, and often utilises quantitative research techniques.

The so-called 'medical model' has become synonymous with reductionism, quantification and physicalism. This is, of course, a very extreme caricature of medicine since many medical writers talk of the art and science of medicine (Sacks, 1982). They note that medicine is a very imperfect science and that medicine has a human and caring focus in the same way that nursing does.

The case of Bob, discussed above, was a rather simplistic comparison of an holistic and a reductionist approach. The difference between these two approaches is that the former is focused upon larger or macroscopic structures. In this example, the focus is upon Bob, a person with feelings, beliefs and relationships with other people. The holistic approach considers context, values and meaning as central features. In contrast, the reductionist approach has a more microscopic perspective: persons, feelings and values are replaced by physical processes, causal relationships and theories of explanation as the more central features.

For the nurse, the holistic approach seems a more appropriate model for practice since the focus of nursing is the whole of the person rather than an isolated aspect of physiology or biochemistry – although these may represent important factors in the nursing care of the person concerned.

So far in this overview, only the concept of reductionism has been considered. Reductionism has been discussed in contrast to holism, hence providing only a negative definition of holism. Something more concrete is required if a positive definition of holism is to be given.

Not all thinkers after Descartes chose to ignore mental substance in favour of physical substance. A distinct European school of thought gradually evolved, which centred on the mental or subjective aspects of experience and ways in which these could be characterised. The German philosopher Immanuel Kant (1724–1804) discussed the way in which the mind of the thinker might influence the way in which the world was perceived. Franz Brentano (1838–1917), the German philosopher and psychologist, attempted to define mental events by the characteristic way in which the mind is directed towards the objects of thought; this he called 'intentionality'.

Under the influence of Descartes, Kant and Brentano, a number of modern philosophers and psychologists contributed to a branch of philosophical enquiry called phenomenology, a technique and theory first developed by Edmund Husserl (1859–1938) and further expanded by his pupil Martin Heidegger (1889–1976). Husserl's contribution to phenomenology was to introduce the phenomenological method and identify the specific area of enquiry for phenomenology, namely the way in which the world presents itself through experience. The phenomenological method requires that one concentrate on the nature of this experience while 'bracketing' or removing oneself from any theoretical beliefs or assumptions that may bias this process.

Heidegger further developed phenomenology by emphasising that being a person cannot be separated from that person's experience of the world, and experience is therefore necessarily 'personified'; hence, any person's experience will be shaped by the very fact of being a person. Phenomenology has had a great influence on contemporary thought, the social sciences generally and nursing in particular (Walters, 1995).

Nursing Practice

One of the most readily recognised philosophical influences on nursing practice can be seen in the work of Benner (1984), who directly acknowledges the influence of phenomenology. Benner's exploration of expertise in nursing attempted to exemplify the expert nurse through examples of expert practice, contrasted at times with novice practice. A tenet of this approach is the idea that the expert 'shows' her expertise in her practice and that this defies further reduction.

Benner develops her account via a taxonomy, that is, a classification of skill. According to this taxonomy, the novice nurse works by following a number of individual rules for practice. These rules are followed rigidly and in relative isolation from other rules; there is no connection between rules, nor flexibility in applying the rules. As the beginner becomes more advanced, the rules are utilised in a much more integrated and complementary way, although they are clearly seen as guiding the behaviour. By the time the nurse becomes an expert, it is as if the nurse has abandoned the rules. The skill of the expert nurse is seamless and flowing, responding spontaneously to the demands of the situation as if by intuition. Benner argues that it is impossible to capture the skill of the expert nurse by reducing that skill to a set of constituent rules for practice: the skill of the expert nurse is holistic.

An analogous example may be useful. Imagine teaching a person how to ride a bicycle by first describing to them how it is done. The description would consist of a series of very detailed instructions, which, if carried out individually, would probably end in disaster. Once the novice rider mounts the bicycle, she will begin to feel how those rules work together to produce the desired effect. With practice, the novice will become competent and eventually expert. The expert cyclist is able to use the bicycle as if it were an extension of her own body, spontaneously responding to new terrain and twists and turns in the road.

The point of referring to the work of Benner is that it provides an example of an overt link with the philosophical heritage discussed above. More than that, Benner attempts to analyse one way in which holism applies to nursing, namely that the skill of the expert nurse is holistic and therefore defies a reductionist description.

Nursing Research

The second major area of influence of holistic/phenomenological thought has been on research methods. Some nurse researchers, following other social scientists, have rejected the quantitative methods of traditional science and adopted phenomenological principles (Holmes, 1990). These researchers argue that reducing the complex phenomenon of human social interactions to measurable components fails to capture the most important elements of the phenomenon. The example of the pillow has shown how it was impossible to capture the important property of 'softness' by a reductionist description. The example of Bob illustrates how the scientific approach failed to capture important aspects of his pain experience and the process of treating it.

Other researchers (for example, Dunlop, 1986) argue that reductionist scientific research into nursing itself fails to capture essential aspects of nursing. A range of other criticisms have been levelled at quantitative research methods. Spencer (1983) argues that utilising quantitative methods in health-care research treats people as objects. Quantitative research relies on statistical analysis so results are expressed in terms of statistical norms, therefore, it is argued, disregarding important individual experiences.

Feminist researchers have been particularly vociferous in their criticisms of quantitative research methods as manipulative, domineering and dismissive of participants as mere subjects (Webb, 1993; Perry, 1994).

So far in this paper, an overview has been given of some of the historical influences on the development of the concept of holism related to nursing. By comparing and contrasting holism and reduc- tionism, the negative definition of holism has been discussed and the foundation for a positive definition established.

In order to take this discussion of holism further, two theories of holism will be defined, utilising comments from nursing literature. The theories will be called the Strong theory and the Weak theory of holism (see below). A degree of latitude should be granted to these definitions, since it is impossible in reality to identify two such clearly demarcated camps within nursing. Nevertheless, this distinction will be used primarily to clarify some of the issues highlighted so far. A secondary intention is that this discussion will provide stimulation for further philosophical research in this area.

HOLISM: THE STRONG THEORY

The Strong theory will take the following definition of holism: things are greater than simply the sum of their constituent parts (cf. Phillips, 1977). Adoption of Strong theory brings at least three implications:

1. The reductionist approach is incompatible with holism (Griffin, 1993).
2. The whole is more than the sum of its parts.
3. The parts cannot be understood if considered in isolation from the whole (Allen, 1991).

Griffin states (1993, p. 310) that 'holism is against all forms of reductionism'. This is the most explicit statement of the Strong theory discovered in a recent survey of the nursing literature. It must be stressed that this is not a claim that Griffin is advocating the Strong theory of holism in her paper; as noted above, no such clearly defined thesis exists. The point is that this remark is just one example of a tendency that implies the Strong theory and, as such, contributes to the problematic nature of this concept.

The problems with the Strong theory of holism stem from the incompatibility of this thesis with other central concepts in nursing and important aspects of nursing practice. Examples from two areas – nursing research and nursing practice – will be considered here before going on to consider the Weak theory of holism.

Strong holism and nursing research

The physical sciences are synonymous with quantitative research methods. The success of these methods of investigation in terms of the discovery and ability to predict through general scientific laws has resulted in the dominance of the physical science model as *the* scientific research method. Nursing has itself been influenced by this model to the extent that the majority of contemporary nursing research is quantitative in nature.

However, there has recently been a growing concern that the model of the physical sciences is incompatible with nursing values (Owen and Holmes, 1993). This concern, although not always explicitly expressed, is with the metaphysical commitments that are implied by the model of the physical sciences. One specific concern is that the quantitative method is reductionist and that this entails a commitment to the view that the world can be described completely by a description of its component parts. This issue was introduced earlier in this chapter, the concern there being that a complex phenomenon such as pain could not be adequately described at the biochemical level. Strong holists argue that to do this would be to miss out completely dimensions of the phenomenon that are central to nursing practice, for example, that pain is not simply an event within a nervous system but a person's experience. Moreover, the effects of the pain may spill over from that person to affect others close to him or her.

The Strong holist takes the view that the model of the physical sciences is not just another useful tool, like a thermometer, but that it is a statement of metaphysical beliefs that are incompatible with the belief in pain as an experience of a person, a person in the social context of family and friends. The positive claim from the Strong holist is that only qualitative research methods should be used by nurse researchers since only these are compatible with the metaphysical assumptions of Strong holism.

The difficulty with the Strong holist view is that it becomes a straitjacket to nursing research and practice. While the limitations of the physical science model are increasingly acknowledged (Guba and

Lincoln, 1994), the Strong holist does not recognise the equally problematic limitations of the qualitative approach.

If nurses were to commit themselves exclusively to qualitative research methods in the belief that these methods alone were compatible with holism, it would be a restrictive and retrograde step for the profession. Restricting nurse researchers to one methodology would limit the range of possible research but might also effect opportunities for collaboration with other disciplines and, on a more practical level, opportunities for funding. This kind of commitment may also compromise the practical role of certain nurses, for example, research nurses, whose collaborative work in large-scale clinical trials arguably can be seen as bringing holistic values to bear in what might otherwise be seen as faceless science. Nursing has had no difficulty in assimilating the beneficial knowledge gained about diseases and their treatment through 'reductionist science' into practice, but how does this fit with a commitment to Strong holism?

Strong holism and nursing practice

According to Strong holism, 'Holism is against all forms of reductionism' (Griffin, 1993, p. 310). When applied to nursing practice, this approach faces a number of difficulties. The Strong holist position, as stated above, claims that the reductionist approach is incompatible with holism, but many aspects of nursing rely, in one form or another, on reductionism. Any system, and nursing operates within the healthcare system, is reductionist in the sense that it is reducible to a set of rule-governed processes.

The nursing process, for example, is itself a means of reducing the care of highly complex individuals to a set of objectives based upon their needs. The very language of 'system' and 'process' presupposes reductionism in the metaphysical sense. Establishing needs and evaluating outcomes may themselves entail quantitative measures: for example, recording vital signs, fluid input and output. Nursing care itself may be directed by the findings of scientific investigations such as biochemical blood results and X-ray investigations. The nursing management of pain relies, in part, on a 'reductionist', scientific understanding of pain and the action of analgesic agents.

The claim that the whole is more than the sum of its parts and that the parts cannot be understood if considered in isolation from the whole (Allen, 1991) is problematic for nursing practice. The problem for the Strong holist here is in showing which 'whole' matters for nursing.

The concept of holism, without any interpretation, is inherently imprecise. Nurses are, at the very least, responsible for their patients, and a patient is a person. But a person is part of a family, part of a society, part of a race. There seems to be no limit to the number of greater 'wholes' to which this individual belongs. So to which 'wholes' do nurses have responsibility?

It must be possible to circumscribe the scope of nursing, to say what nursing is and is not, to state the limits of an individual nurse's responsibilities. Patient allocation could itself be described as reductionist, yet the patient is, in most instances, the main focus of nursing care. In practice, nurses recognise the limits to their own practice, 'liaison' and 'referral' being part of the language of nursing.

The Strong holist may reply that individual nurses are responsible to their patients and that nursing is responsible to the greater whole. However, rather than clarifying the dispute, this only adds to the vagueness of holism. The Strong holist must be able to reconcile the demands of Strong holism with the demands of a profession committed to practice and research within a multiprofessional framework. At the very least, the Strong theory of holism would render nursing impossible; how could one nurse meet these demands? What would happen to the concept of multidisciplinary care? These are the types of question that a nurse committed to Strong holism must be able to answer.

HOLISM: THE WEAK THEORY

The Weak theory of holism is less a reaction to reductionism and more an attempt to create a positive definition of holism. Again, it must be highlighted that the Weak theory of holism is not advocated by an identifiable camp within nursing but is implicit in the practice of nurse clinicians and the discussions of nurse researchers and scholars. The Weak holist recognises the significance of the parts/whole relationship and the importance of context for defining the particular 'whole' that is significant for nursing.

For many nurses, the significant whole to which their care is directed is the individual person, the patient. This view is adjusted according to context to cover other significant wholes, for example, the patient's family or society. The infection control nurse may be concerned with the manifestations of an infectious illness within one person, but this concern may soon extend to care for a family or the whole of a community for which this infection may have implications.

For the nurse who is a ward manager, the significant whole will be the entire ward, patients and staff included. The fact that the manager delegates aspects of the work to several individuals is reductionist in the sense that it recognises that there are discrete areas of work to be attended to, but as a means of maintaining the integrity of the whole. There is no inherent contradiction with holism.

Weak holism and research

Weak holism recognises the importance of quantitative methods of research because they provide an effective means of inquiry into holistic structures, be they individual people, groups of people or wider structures. Qualitative methods are used in situations where quantitative methods have limited application. The reductionism required by quantitative methods is not sensitive to individuals, to contexts, to meaning or to values that are important to a profession whose focus is on the care of people. This does not mean that the results of quantitative research have no place; physics, biochemistry and mechanics all have their place as foundations to inform holistic practice.

Guba and Lincoln (1994, p. 116) recommend a 'continuing dialogue' between researchers who use either method, both within nursing and between disciplines. The use of triangulation methods (Carr, 1994), the evaluation of the strengths and weaknesses of each approach to an area of research, is a positive if pragmatic dialogue. There needs also to be dialogue of a more philosophical nature if the metaphysical assumptions of each approach are to be made commensurable.

One positive move would be for nurse researchers to be trained in a range of research methods. Nurse researchers should not be made to feel that they have compromised their commitment to holism by utilising a range of research methods:

> Thus nurses, for example, can research areas of knowledge that are likely to be useful to them in caring, following patterns that have been laid down in public health, epidemiology, physiology, biology, psychology and social psychology, to mention those disciplines which seem most central to their focus. Nursing-caring may determine the questions, but conceptualisation and methodologies are borrowed from the established disciplines. (Dunlop, 1986, pp. 665–6)

Weak holism and practice

Weak holism is compatible with all aspects of nursing practice since it emphasises the focus of care, the whole of the person, within the most significant context. The context may be defined by practical factors, for example, the context and setting in which the person presents as a patient. Weak holism is practically compatible with reductionist science because scientific fact – blood cell count, electrolyte balance, principles of wound healing, mechanisms of drug action – provide a foundation on which holistic practice is often based.

Scientific facts frequently provide the rationale for individual differences in care between patients. In the example of Bob's pain, it was argued that the reductionist account of Approach 1 could be assimilated into the holistic account of Approach 2 but that the reverse could not occur. In Approach 1, the focus of care (Bob), and the context of care (Bob's pain, his cancer, his relationship with his family) are lost.

The holistic nature of Approach 2 puts the focus of care at the appropriate level for nursing, which also utilises knowledge of the pain mechanism and drug action to provide appropriate care. Nurses can combine and move between the different demands made upon them as researchers, educators, clinicians and carers to patients and their families. Weak holism is compatible with this necessary flexibility.

CONCLUSION

This chapter introduces the problem of defining the concept of holism in nursing. A philosophical approach has been taken in exploring some of the issues in this complex debate. A limited review of some of the historical influences that have informed this debate within nursing has been given. Two theories of holism are defined – Strong holism and Weak holism – as a means of suggesting a way forward in defining the concept of holism in a manner compatible with nursing practice and research. It was argued that, if holism is defined only negatively, in terms of its opposition to reductionism, nurses are forced towards the Strong holism camp, which becomes self-defeating. 'Holism', like any other concept, has a meaning that has evolved and will continue to evolve over time. Nurses must continue to attempt to positively define this concept if it is to remain central to nursing.

REFERENCES

Allen, C.E. (1991) An analysis of the pragmatic consequences of holism for nursing, *Western Journal of Nursing Research*, **13**(2): 256–72.

Benner, P. (1984) *From Novice to Expert* (London: Addison-Wesley).

Carr, L.T. (1994) The strengths and weaknesses of quantitative and qualitative research: what method for nursing?, *Journal of Advanced Nursing*, **20**: 716–21.

Cribb, A., Bignold, S. and Ball, S.J. (1994) Linking the parts: an exemplar of philosophical and practical issues in holistic nursing, *Journal of Advanced Nursing*, **20**: 233–8.

Descartes, R. (1977, trans. F.E. Sutcliffe) *Discourse on Method and Meditations* (London: Penguin).

Dunlop, M.J. (1986) Is a science of caring possible?, *Journal of Advanced Nursing*, **11**: 661–70.

Griffin, A. (1993) Holism in nursing: its meaning and value, *British Journal of Nursing*, **2**(6): 310–12.

Guba, E.G. and Lincoln, Y.S. (1994) Competing paradigms in qualitative research, in Denzin, N.K. and Lincoln, Y.S. (eds) pp. 105–17 *Handbook of Qualitative Research* (London: Sage).

Ham-Ying, S. (1993) Analysis of the concept of holism within the context of nursing, *British Journal of Nursing*, **2**(15): 771–5.

Harre, R. (1989) *The Philosophies of Science* (Oxford: Oxford University Press).

Holmes, C.A. (1990) Alternatives to natural science foundations for nursing, *International Journal of Nursing Studies*, **27**(3): 187–98.

Jacono, J.B. and Jacono J.J. (1994) How should holism guide the setting of educational standards?, *Journal of Advanced Nursing*, **19**: 342–6.

Kolcaba, K.Y. (1992) A taxonomic structure for the concept comfort, *Image: Journal of Nursing Scholarship*, **23**(4): 237–40.

Kolcaba, K.Y. (1994) A theory of holistic comfort for nursing, *Journal of Advanced Nursing*, **19**: 1178–84.

Liaschenko, J. and Davis, A.J. (1991) Nurses and physicians on nutritional support: a comparision, *Journal of Medicine and Philosophy*, **16**(3): 259–83.

Owen, M.J. and Holmes, C.A. (1993) 'Holism' in the discourse of nursing, *Journal of Advanced Nursing*, **18**: 1688–95.

Perry, P. (1994) Feminist empiricism as a method for inquiry in nursing, *Western Journal of Nursing*, **16**(5): 480–94.

Phillips, D.C. (1977) *Holistic Thought in Social Science* (California: Stanford University Press).

Rogers, M. (1970) *An Introduction to the Theoretical Basis of Nursing* (Philadelphia: FA Davis).

Rogers, M. (1980) Nursing: a science of unitary man, in Riehl, J. and Roy, C., (eds) *Conceptual Models for Nursing Practice*, 2nd edn, pp. 329–37 (Norwalk, CT: Appleton-Century-Crofts).

Sacks, O. (1982) *Awakenings* (London: Pan).

Sarter, B. (1988) Philosophical sources of nursing theory, *Nursing Science Quarterly*, **1**(2): 52–9.

Smuts, J.C. (1926) *Holism and Evolution* (New York: Macmillan).

Spencer, J. (1983) Research with the human touch, *Nursing Times*, **29**(12): 24–7.

Walters, A. (1995) The phenomenological movement: implications for nursing research, *Journal of Advanced Nursing*, **22**: 791–9.

Watson, J. (1985) *Nursing, Human Science and Human Care: A Theory of Nursing* (Norwalk, CT: Appleton-Century-Crofts).

Webb, C. (1993) Feminist research: definitions, methodology, methods and evaluation, *Journal of Advanced Nursing*, **18**: 416–23.

CHAPTER FIVE

Positivism as a method in nursing research

EDITOR'S INTRODUCTION

This chapter tries, first of all, to make clear what positivism is. Then an attempt is made to show why positivism is deeply unsuited to much nursing research. The reasons stem partly from the fact that a great deal of nursing research centres on the mental states of patients and clients, or nurses themselves. The chapter aims to show that the objects of such enquiries seem, in principle, impossible to capture with only the conceptual resources that the positivist permits.

Positivism as a method
in nursing research

Steven Edwards

Very roughly, positivism is a scientific method, a proposed, systematic way of finding out about things or, more grandly, of discovering empirical facts. Nursing research, of course, involves an attempt to find things out – just as scientific research is such an attempt.

It is evident that the majority of nurse theorists and researchers do not think positivism to be a suitable method for employment in nursing research (Benner, 1985, 1994; Kikuchi and Simmons, 1992). It is less evident just why this is so, and it is not clear, in rejecting positivism, just what it is that is being rejected. One commentator, Halfpenny, claims to identify 12 varieties of positivism (1982, pp. 114–17). So, in being 'opposed to Positivism', it is far from clear just what it is that one is opposed to. In what follows, an attempt is made to identify the main characteristics of positivism and to show why it is a research method unsuited to the subject matter of much nursing research.

HALFPENNY'S DOZEN VARIETIES OF POSITIVISM

Auguste Comte (1788–1857) is widely regarded as the official founder of positivism. His intention seems to have been to apply to social science, the methods that appeared to be generating great success in natural science. The term 'positivism' is apparently intended to indicate that positivists will only accept that which is 'positively true' so to speak, or which has a '"positive" basis' (Oldroyd, 1986, p. 170).

According to Halfpenny, Comte can be associated with at least four of the 12 versions of positivism he identifies. Positivism 1 amounts to a thesis concerning the development of human thought such that it involves a transition from theological to metaphysical to positive phases. Crudely, it is suggested that this transition represents a progression in human thought. It is a progression from the employment of primitive, mystical explanations to sophisticated scientific

91

explanations. Positivism 2 is the view that sensory evidence provides the ground for all genuine knowledge. Positivism 3 is the thesis that all the disciplines that seek to extend human knowledge should employ the same method. This has been termed the 'Unity of Science' thesis, or for obvious reasons, 'methodological monism'. Positivism 4 emerged in Comte's later work. This is described by Halfpenny as 'a secular religion of humanity devoted to the worship of society' (1982, pp. 19–20). It is worth adding that Positivism 4 is regarded as untypical of positivist thought and even to conflict with certain of Comte's own views. Indeed, Halfpenny describes Positivism 4 as 'an aberration' (1982).

Positivism 5 is ascribed by Halfpenny to Spencer (1820–1903). This is a view according to which societies progress as a consequence of the competition between the individuals who compose them. It is described as an 'evolutionary theory of history' by Halfpenny (1982, p. 22). As in evolutionary theory, the suggestion is that societies are developments and improvements upon earlier forms. This is related in some respects to Positivism 1.

Durkheim (1858–1917) is described as a proponent of Positivism 6 by Halfpenny. This is a thesis according to which knowledge of society stems from collections of facts and from statistical analyses of these. This is the method employed in Durkheim's classic study of suicide (Durkheim, 1952).

Positivisms 7, 8, 9 and 10 are closely related and can be assimilated for our purposes. They involve the views of that group of philosophers and scientists known as the logical positivists. Roughly, they put forward a verificationist theory of meaning in which scientific terms or expression are meaningful only if they derive from some verifiable sensory experience. Thus, the meaning of term 'red' derives from its association with sensory experiences of red things. Furthermore, these four versions of positivism seek to outline a formal structure for the scientific enterprise. That is, it is supposed that scientific explanations and predictions will share the same overall form (see below). Thus, in this collection of positivist theses – 7, 8, 9 and 10 – a criterion of meaning for scientific terms and theories is proposed, as is a view of the formal structure of scientific explanations.

Positivism 11 is ascribed by Halfpenny (1982, p. 92) to Bacon (1561–1626). It is a view of scientific method according to which scientific laws are derived from particular observations. Finally, Popper is associated with Positivism 12. In this, scientific method involves the putting forward of hypotheses and attempts to show them to be false (Halfpenny, 1982, p. 115).

MAIN FEATURES OF POSITIVISM

An indication of the overall tenor of the group of theses Halfpenny describes can be gleaned. A first feature (1) concerns the emphasis on confirmation or falsification. A second (2) is the weight and importance attached to evidence provided by the senses. A third (3) is the commitment to methodological monism (the view that all disciplines which seek to extend human knowledge should employ the same methods) (cf. Oldroyd, 1986, p. 168). Finally a feature (4), which is, perhaps, neglected in Halfpenny's discussion, is the view that science is value-free (that is, it is neutral in terms of ideological or moral viewpoints).

At first sight, it seems plausible to adopt each of these features if one is intending to obtain knowledge about the world. For example, suppose one wants to discover how best to treat pressure sores. If one wants to know this, one is engaged in research, as one wants to discover something about the nature of the world. Consider the first feature of positivist method just identified. It seems reasonable to require that any claims one makes with regard to a 'best treatment' for pressure sores should be testable. It should be possible to show whether or not one's proposed treatment works. So this first constraint on theorising that is a feature of positivist method seems entirely reasonable: claims made should be open to confirmation or falsification.

The second main feature is related to the first. The requirement that claims can be confirmed or shown to be false raises the question of how confirmation or falsity is to be determined. This second requirement stipulates that the 'court', so to speak, of assessment of theories is sensory evidence: what one can see, hear, touch and so on. Consider the pressure sore example again. In order to confirm or falsify a claim that a specific quantity of a particular drug successfully treats pressure sores, one would, presumably, need to look at a patient who has a pressure sore and who has taken the specified quantity of the relevant drug. In doing this, one is using one's senses in order to assess the plausibility or otherwise of an empirical claim. Moreover, it is worth emphasising that the view that evidence gleaned from the senses, such as sight, is crucial to our obtaining knowledge about the world seems clearly to be highly plausible. Also, the suggestion that such observations provide a foundation of our knowledge of the world seems equally plausible.

The third feature of positivism mentioned above was a commitment to methodological monism. As noted, this is the view that all those researchers who are seeking to extend human knowledge –

natural scientists, social scientists, nursing researchers and so on – should deploy the same method. The reason for this is quite straight-forward. As mentioned above, positivism can be described as a method for discovering facts, for finding out about the world. It is put forward by its proponents as the best method to adopt in the enterprise of discovering facts. Given this, it follows that any discipline that has the aim of discovering facts should adopt those strategies advocated in positivism. Specifically, such disciplines should adopt features 1 and 2 identified above. Moreover, as became evident in our discussion of 'Halfpenny's dozen', requirements 1 and 2 relate to a more general conception of scientific explanation. According to the conception – represented in Positivisms 7, 8, 9 and 10 – scientific explanations have a specific formal structure, roughly the form of an argument that contains two premises and a conclusion. The first premise describes the relevant features of the situation; these are sometimes described as the antecedent conditions. The second premise describes the relevant law of nature, and the conclusion describes the event to be explained or predicted.

Consider the following example:

Premise i (antecedent conditions): The air temperature falls below 0°C.

Premise ii (description of relevant law of nature): Water expands when it freezes.

Conclusion (event to be explained or predicted): My car radiator has burst (explanation) [or will burst (prediction)].

This schema provides an example of scientific explanation. The idea is that premises i and ii serve to explain why my car radiator has burst. As noted, the same form of explanation can also be employed in the prediction of events. Part of the appeal of this model of explanation is that the relationship between the premises and the conclusion is one of necessity. That is, given that premises i and ii are true, the conclusion follows necessarily (provided, of course that the premises are taken together with some supplementary assumptions, for example, that my car is outside in the freezing temperatures, that the radiator is filled to the brim with water, and the truth of natural laws regarding the pres-sure that metal can withstand before bursting).

The fourth and last main feature to be mentioned here concerns the value-neutrality of science. Crudely, the project of finding out about the world should not be polluted by prejudices and commitments to cherished beliefs, nor in fact, by any presuppositions at all. One should be prepared to accept whatever conclusions are thrown up by application of methods 1 and 2 even if they conflict with strongly held beliefs. For example, one might justly be suspicious of research showing that treatment X successfully treated pressure sores if that research were conducted by the manufacturers of treatment X. They would have a clear vested interest in establishing treatment X, so it may be said that their research is not 'value-free' or unbiased. For positivists, commitment to a particular set of values or ideology should be jettisoned for the purposes of conducting research. As with features 1, 2 and 3, this seems a wholly reasonable requirement.

We now have a very brief summary of four of the features that, it is being suggested here, characterise positivism. What I propose to do now is to try to give an indication of the difficulty in applying this method in nursing research.

FIRST- AND THIRD-PERSON PERSPECTIVES

It may be recalled that part of the positivist thesis is the view that all those disciplines which seek to extend human knowledge should employ the same method; this was described as the thesis of methodological monism. Clearly then, positivism supposes that the same methods that are successful in the natural sciences can legitimately and fruitfully be applied in the human sciences. The presupposition is that the study of phenomena such as rocks, planets and tides need not be considered different in kind from the study of humans. The same method – positivist method – can be applied in either field.

However, there is, of course, an important difference between the objects of the natural sciences (physics, geology and so on) and the objects of the human sciences (psychology, sociology, economics and so on). The fact is that humans have minds but planets, rocks and tides do not. So, while it is the case that planets (and so on) have no point of view on what happens to them, or on their situation, this is not the case with humans. They have a point of view, or perspective, from which they see things. This raises at least two serious problems in terms of the appropriateness of positivist method for the study of human beings. The first derives from the fact that humans have 'free will', while rocks and planets do not. The second problem arises from the fact that persons seem to have a unique means of access to their own mental states.

Problem 1: Free Will

The fact that humans have free will has serious ramifications for the explanatory model described above. As we saw, explanations (and predictions) of events are, in that model, couched in the form of an argument with premises and a conclusion. The success of the model in providing explanations depends upon the nature of the relationship between the premises and the conclusion. This is taken to be one of logical necessity; that is to say, if the premises are true (and the laws of nature remain constant), the conclusion *necessarily* follows.

It is, however, not at all clear that such a model could apply in the explanation of human actions. Humans have free will, so, in principle, it appears that there could be no 'law' or generalisation relating to human action that could have the same logical force as a law or generalisation relating to natural phenomena (planets, tides and so on). As we saw earlier in the car radiator example, given the antecedent conditions and the truth of the natural laws, it is necessarily the case that my radiator will burst. However, the task of trying to construct laws that apply to human action seems extremely difficult, if not hopeless. Even a generalisation such as 'Humans eat when hungry and have food available to them' has numerous exceptions. Hunger-strikers, persons on religious fasts, those on strict diets and people with anorexia nervosa all provide counterexamples to the suggested 'law'. So if it is accepted that no laws could be posited that determine human action (in the same way in which natural laws determine planetary orbits and so on), no explanations of human action will be forthcoming from the explanatory model posited in positivism and which is supposed essential to any genuinely scientific activity.

Problem 2: Mental States

The second problem can be brought out by distinguishing between two methodological perspectives: the third-person and the first-person. It seems clear that the appropriate methodological perspective from which to study inanimate objects is the third-person perspective. This is the perspective from which things are 'open to view'. Physical changes are plainly open to view in the sense that their occurrence can be witnessed by any number of observers. Hence, the shape of a rock, the flow of a tide and the orbit of a planet are all open to view in a way congenial to the application of positivism. It should be added that physical changes in humans are similarly open to view: pressure sores, changes in temperature, blood pressure are each types of physical change accessible from the third-person perspective. Descriptions of such changes can be confirmed or falsified by those other than the person who has the pressure sore, the high temperature or the high blood pressure. Such phenomena are open to view and so are accessible from the third-person perspective – the perspective of people other than the person whose condition is being described.

However, it does not follow from the fact that the third-person perspective is the most appropriate for the study of inanimate objects, that it is the most appropriate for the study of humans (specifically, things which have minds). The reason is obvious. Positivist method emphasises the importance of confirmation and falsifiability. These are virtues of theoretical claims in positivism. However, it seems that important parts of the mental lives of humans are essentially private to the person concerned. A great many, perhaps all, mental states are privately experienced. They occur in the mind of the person who experiences or thinks them. So such mental states seem, at least, not to be open to view in the way, for example, that the movements of the tides are open to view. It thus seems that humans have available to them a perspective on their own mental states which is unique to them and which no other person can adopt: the first-person perspective.

Moreover, it seems to be the case that the first-person perspective on mental states is a particularly special one. It is considered that a person currently thinking is in a privileged position when it comes to determining just what it is that is being thought. This is the phenomenon of privileged access (Hamlyn, 1970). Thus, it seems problematic to accommodate the scientific study of mental states (thoughts, sensations, emotions) from the positivist perspective. Positivism seeks to anchor research findings in the observable, in that which is indisputably evident, in data such as the movement of a tide or the freezing of water. Confirmation or falsification of claims made about these kinds of phenomenon can be made from the third-person perspective, but when it comes to research into the mental states of humans, at least two kinds of problem arise.

First (A) is that there is, apparently, a range of data that, it seems, is accessible to one person only: the person who actually experiences the relevant mental states. Of course, the person might choose to reveal to others just what it is that he is thinking or feeling, but also he might not. So, in principle, there appears to be a range of data beyond the reach of the third-person perspective.

Second (B), it seems that that person is the person best placed to determine the nature of those states. For example, if we ask him questions such as 'What are you thinking?', 'What are you feeling?' or 'Are you in pain?', it appears that he is in the best position to provide an answer to that question. How might the positivist respond to these problems?

TWO POSITIVIST RESPONSES TO PROBLEM 2

Behaviourism

One response to problems A and B is simply to tailor mental states to suit positivist method. That is, one might try to argue that mental states are best construed in such a way that they are accessible from the third-person perspective – are open to view. One may do this by advocating a crude form of behaviourism. One may claim that mental states are to be identified with behaviour and thus assert that mental states simply *are* behaviours. In such a view, pain would simply equate with pain behaviour. A desire for a drink of water would be identical with water-seeking behaviour.

This strategy copes with problem A since the realm of privately accessible phenomena has now been made public: mental states are behavioral states and these are open to view in the way in which positivist method requires. The strategy also copes with problem B. Since a person's behaviours are open to view, and these are to be identified with his mental states, the thinker cannot now claim privileged access to his own mental states so cannot legitimately claim to be authoritative with respect to what he is thinking, feeling. The reason is that he is no longer in a privileged position to determine what it is that he is thinking or feeling. Since his mental states are open to view, the thinker is in the same position as everyone else when it comes to determining just what it is that he is thinking or feeling.

Problems with the behaviourist solution

Although the option of behaviourism might solve the problems for the positivist that are generated by problems A and B, the behaviourist thesis itself seems vulnerable to some serious criticisms.[1] In short, as may be expected, the attempt to tailor mental states to suit positivist method seems open to serious objection. For example, it seems to be part of the very concept of pain that it is something one *experiences*.

There seems such a great distance between the experience of pain and pain behaviours that it is implausible merely to identify these. It is plain that a person may be in pain but may keep this to himself – may suffer in silence – and may not behave in any way indicating that he is experiencing pain. So pain behaviour seems not to be a plausible necessary condition of pain. Also, it is evident that a person may merely pretend to be in pain without actually being in pain: actors do this all the time. Thus, it is clear that pain behaviour is not even a sufficient condition of pain since a person may simply be acting. Thus, this strategy for resolving the problems that mental states generate for positivist method seems not to be successful, and the problems remain. The apparent 'privacy' of mental states means they are resistant to study conducted exclusively from the third-person perspective.

Mind–brain identity theory

A second positivist response is to identify mental states not with behaviours but with neurological states (cf. Armstrong, 1968). This is a position that has seemed attractive to many philosophers in the 20th century.[2] In this strategy, problem A is defeated because, in principle, it would be possible to determine just what a person is thinking simply by examining his brain. Of course, this requires that much more is known about the brain than is presently known, but this, it may be said, is not a forlorn hope: neuroscience is progressing at a rapid rate.

This strategy is also able to overcome problem B because the person does not now have a privileged access to his own mental states. In principle, it is possible for others to 'read off' what he is thinking from examination of his neurological states. So, as in the behaviourist strategy, the asymmetry between the perspective of the thinker on his own mental states and the perspective of others on those states is undermined. With the undermining of this asymmetry, privileged access is also undermined. So this is, perhaps, a more promising strategy for the positivist to adopt than the behaviourist one.

Problems with mind–brain identity theory

However, this thesis too has been shown to be vulnerable to quite serious objection.[3] It is not important for us to go through some of the more technical of the criticisms to which this thesis has been subjected. However, two criticisms can be given quite quickly. The first centres on sensation states, and the second on thoughts. The first criticism asserts that the relationship held to obtain between mental and neurological states in mind–brain identity theory is implausibly rigid. It is suggested that, according to the theory, mental states of one type – for example, pain states – are identified with a type of neurological states; let us call these N-states. But, the objection runs, it is perfectly possible that there may be persons, or non-humans, who experience pain states in the absence of their having N-states; perhaps, instead of N-states, such persons are found to have O-states or P-states. This objection thus queries the claimed intimacy of the relations between types of mental and neurological state that is advanced in mind–brain identity theory.

A second criticism is again one that queries the intimacy of the relationship between mental and neurological states. This objection suggests that, in order to know what a person thinks, it could never be enough simply to examine his neurological states. It would be necessary to know something of the person's environment, to know what language he speaks, what his culture is like and so on (see Edwards, 1994).

As noted, I will not give these matters any extended discussion. My intention is simply to indicate two of the possible responses to problems A and B that are available to positivists and to signal some of the difficulties with each of the responses.[4]

WHY SEEK AN ALTERNATIVE TO POSITIVISM?

A common criticism of the medical enterprise, is that it regards patients as objects rather than as people, that is, individuals with a point of view (Liaschenko and Davis, 1991). It assumes that patients are more like rocks and planets than individuals who undergo mental experiences. In short, the criticism is that the medical enterprise has attempted to apply positivist methodology to human subjects and that this has led to an impoverishment in the implementation of health care. Proponents of such a critique of the medical enterprise typically point to the fact that this impoverishment is recognised in the nursing literature and that nurses are particularly conscious of it. The suggestion is that the medical enterprise can be charged with placing too great an emphasis on the third-person perspective and of neglecting to take into account the importance of the first-person perspective.

It is commonly pointed out that there is a way it *feels* to be ill and that this 'feeling' aspect of illness – sometimes described as the phenomenological aspect of illness – is part of the way in which illness is understood (Cassell, 1991). For example, it is plausible to suppose that there is more to influenza than the objective signs associated with it. There seems to be more to the concepts of illness and disease than is accessible from the third-person perspective, specifically, the 'feeling' or phenomenological aspect of illness. Moreover, this 'feeling' or phenomenological aspect of illness is clearly quite central to health care and its implementation. One person, A, might have a high temperature but feel relatively well. Another, person B, might have the same temperature but feel dreadful. Thus, even though the two people appear to be in the same state when this is assessed from the third-person perspective (for example, the same temperature and same blood pressure), the way in which they experience their illness is significantly different. One feels devastated and wrecked; the other feels only moderately ill.

Hence, factors accessible, it appears, *only* from the first-person perspective – the perspective of the sufferer – seem so essential to our understanding of illness that any research into health care would need to take such factors into account. Indeed, for at least some types of research, the inclusion of such factors would appear to be absolutely essential. From the point of view of nursing research, then, it would seem to be the case that the kind of data that are unique to the first-person perspective are exactly the kind of data that need to be enquired into, as it is this range of data which is crucial to the experiences of illness, of being cared for and of being a carer.

The importance of this range of data is reflected in the research projects taken on by nurse researchers. These include how it feels to experience a particular illness, how it feels to be nursed, how it feels to experience moral conflicts in one's work, how users of mental health services perceive nurses and so on. Such research projects seek to describe the experiences from the perspective of the person who experiences them – the perspective of the research subject. They are attempts to bring out into the open and to elucidate data that seems inaccessible, namely, the mental states of subjects, their perceptions, feelings and emotions.

Given agreement that many nurse researchers seek to enquire into data that are tied to the first-person perspective, the problem arises of how to obtain these data and, of course, of how to interpret the data once they are obtained. This last difficulty – that relating to interpretation of data – leads on to a deeper criticism of positivism than those considered here so far.

A 'DEEPER' CRITICISM

Criticisms of the attempt to apply positivist method to the human sciences have been levelled at the positivist enterprise by a number of philosophers, notably, Winch (1958) and Heidegger (1962). It is fair to say that these criticisms have been taken up by a number of nurse theorists (Benner, 1994). Very crudely, the criticism suggests that explanations of human action necessarily involve appeal to 'reasonableness' or rationality. In order to explain a human action, it will be necessary to determine how a person conceives of, or interprets, his predicament, for it is on the basis of such interpretations that persons act.

The notion of interpretation is crucial also for the researcher who is seeking to explain the actions or feelings of her subjects, as a single set of behaviours can be interpreted in an indefinite number of ways. For example, suppose a person leaves a room. This may have a wide number of explanations, each depending upon how the behaviour is interpreted by the researcher. The person may have left the room owing to feelings of embarrassment or boredom, or he may have wanted to indicate displeasure at what was occurring in the room, and so on. This problem of interpretation does not seem paralleled in the natural sciences. Explanations of the behaviour of, for example, planets are plainly not dependent on their intentions because they do not have minds.

Thus, in order to explain a human action, it seems necessary to determine how it is rational to act by the actor's own lights, more grandly, to determine which criteria of rationality are applied by the person whose actions are to be explained. This presents a further set of problems as one's views regarding what counts as rational seem to be largely determined by one's own cultural heritage and upbringing. For example, suppose one is invited to continue the following series of numbers: '2, 4, 6, 8...'. It seems rational to continue this by the series '10, 12, 14, 16...'. But suppose it is claimed that the correct way, the rational way, to continue is to repeat the first four numbers and so have a series like this: '2, 4, 6, 8, 2, 4, 6, 8, 10, 12, 14, 16, 10, 12, 14, 16...'. The second option seems odd, but it would be harsh to judge it irrational. There is an intelligible sequence being followed, if not the one which seemed natural for us to follow, 'natural', that is, by our standards of what is rational.

So this deeper objection to the application of positivist method indicates a crucial role for interpretation in the explanation of human action and in responses to situations. The need for interpretation of action in their explanation raises further difficulties concerning what is to count as rational. These complications cause problems for positivist method since they suggest that the facts of a situation cannot simply be read off from an observation of it. That is, human actions are not 'open to view' in the way that positivism requires as they are partly constituted by the human agent's interpretation of situations in which they act. Explanations of such actions thus seem required to take the agent's perspective into account, and this, it seems, is not simply open to view.

It should be added that the difficulties we have just noted in accounting for human action arise for any proposed method seeking to explain or understand human action – including so-called hermeneutic or interpretivist methods. One such method, which fully appreciates the difficulties just mentioned and which proposes ways around them, is that of interpretive phenomenology (Benner, 1994). However, I shall not attempt any discussion of that method. I will draw this paper to a close by reiterating the point regarding the centrality of the concept of interpretation in relation to the health-care context.

Benner and Wrubel (1989, p. 58) suggest that 'background meanings and personal concerns actually set up what counts as "stressful"'. Put differently, their suggestion is that the interpretation by a patient of a situation as stressful derives from an interpretation of the situation by the patient and that this will be determined, in part, by previous interpretations of situations experienced by the patient.

To press this further, consider questions such as 'How are you?' and 'How are you feeling?' Answers to these questions cannot be read off from objective signs. The patient's answer will be rooted in an interpretation of his predicament, and this interpretation will, in turn, not be independent of the patient's own self-interpretations, by which it is meant, for example, the patient's own views concerning the kind of person he is and the kind of person he wants to be. For example, suppose the patient regards himself as a highly independent man and values his independence extremely highly. If his interpretation of illness is that this independence will be severely compromised, it is reasonable to suppose that the impact of the illness on him will be very great. Moreover, an appreciation of this significance by his carers would seem to be very important. The example is supposed to indicate that interpretation pervades health-care work (see especially Benner and Wrubel, 1989). Patients and clients whom nurses encounter interpret their predicaments, as, of course, do nurses themselves. This suggests that situations are at least partly constituted by the significance or meaning accorded to the situation by those within it. Since these various shades of significance cannot simply be read off from the situation, and since it is these which are plausibly regarded as the concern of nurse researchers, it appears that positivist method is not appropriate for nurse research.

NOTES

1. It should be said that there are at least three versions of behaviourism: metaphysical, methodological and analytical (see Flew, 1979, pp. 39–40).
2. For a critical survey, see Macdonald (1989).
3. More strictly, it is being supposed here that type–type identities are the kind required by the positivist, and it will be claimed that such theories are open to strong objection. Of course, token–token identity theories need not be considered vulnerable to the same objections. For an account of these technicalities, see Macdonald (1989).
4. Those who wish to pursue these matters are referred to Macdonald (1989).

REFERENCES

Armstrong, D.M. (1968) *A Materialist Theory of Mind* (London: Routledge & Kegan Paul).

Benner, P. (1985) Quality of life: a phenomenological perspective on explanation, prediction, and understanding in nursing science, *Advances in Nursing Science*, **8**(1): 1–14.

Benner, P (ed.) (1994) *Interpretive Phenomenology* (London: Sage).

Benner, P. and Wrubel, J. (1989) *The Primacy of Caring* (Menlo Park, CA: Addison-Wesley).

Cassell, E.J. (1991) *The Nature of Suffering* (Oxford: Oxford University Press).

Durkheim, E. (1952) *Suicide, a Study in Sociology* (London: Routledge & Kegan Paul).

Edwards, S.D. (1994) *Externalism in the Philosophy of Mind* (Aldershot: Avebury).

Flew, A. (1979) *A Dictionary of Philosophy* (London: Pan).

Halfpenny, P. (1982) *Positivism and Sociology* (London: George Allen & Unwin).

Hamlyn, D.W. (1970) *The Theory of Knowledge* (London: Macmillan).

Heidegger, M. (1962, trans. J. Macquarrie and E. Robinson) *Being and Time* (Oxford: Blackwell).

Kikuchi, J.F. and Simmons, H. (eds) (1992) *Philosophic Inquiry in Nursing* (London: Sage).

Liaschenko, J. and Davis, A.J. (1991) Nurses and physicians on nutritional support: a comparison, *Journal of Medicine and Philosophy*, **16**: 259–83.

Macdonald, C. (1989) *Mind–Body Identity Theories* (London: Routledge).

O'Hear, A. (1990) *An Introduction to the Philosophy of Science* (Oxford: Oxford University Press).

Oldroyd, D. (1986) *The Arch of Knowledge* (London: Methuen).

Winch, P. (1958) *The Idea of a Social Science* (London: Routledge & Kegan Paul).

CHAPTER SIX

Towards a credible theory
of mind for nursing

EDITOR'S INTRODUCTION

Edward Lepper's chapter tries to shed some light on the problem of what a theory of mind for nursing should look like. He claims that any such theory must be credible from the following four perspectives: the nursing perspective, the scientific perspective, the perspective of 'common sense' and the philosophical perspective.

Cartesian dualism (the theory favoured by Holden, 1991) is rejected on the grounds that it is not credible from the scientific or philosophical perspective. Another theory of mind, materialism, is shown vulnerable to criticism owing to its inadequacy from the perspectives of common sense, philosophy and nursing. A Heideggerian view, favoured by Benner and Wrubel (1989), is rejected due to inadequacy when viewed from a scientific perspective.

Edward Lepper also considers a position explored elsewhere by Paul Dawson (1994), known as emergent materialism. While features of Dawson's approach are viewed sympathetically, his own favoured view is rejected by Lepper on the grounds of inadequacy from the philosophical, scientific and commonsense perspectives. A view championed by Searle (1992) – biological naturalism – is tentatively advanced by Edward Lepper as being a plausible theory of mind for nursing. This theory, he argues, most adequately meets the requirements identified above.

Towards a credible theory of mind for nursing

Edward Lepper

Philosophers have traditionally devoted a great deal of attention to the nature of mind and its relationship to the body, such that the philosophy of mind remains the most actively researched part of the subject. Increasingly, this area is also becoming one of interest and concern to members of the nursing profession. This has come about through increased reflection by nurses on the nature of their work and by developments such as increased specialism, the pursuit of holistic care, changes in nurse education and the evolution of roles within the health-care professions.

A glance at any text in the philosophy of mind will discover references to the 'mind–body problem', which has fuelled several centuries of debate within this area. It remains, however, a good, if well-trodden, way in and a means of illustrating and contrasting theoretical positions, of which there are a vast number. The traditional debate has involved two broad types of theory, namely *dualism* on the one hand and *materialism* (also related to and sometimes equated with *physicalism* or *naturalism*) on the other, although there are many variations on both themes. These two views in particular have been taken up by recent nursing theorists, who have argued that they provide a tenable foundation for nursing practice. Meanwhile, nursing has also drawn theoretical inspiration from continental philosophy, so it is appropriate briefly to contrast this with the analytic (traditionally Anglo-American) perspectives already mentioned. These positions will be explored below, with the intention of providing an introduction, with reference to examples from nursing practice, to the issue of which features a credible theory of mind for nursing should incorporate.

WHAT A CREDIBLE THEORY OF MIND MUST DO

A theory of mind (of the nature of mind and the relation of mind to body) that will provide a solid foundation for nursing practice, theory

109

and research must be acceptable not only to nursing, but also to science, philosophy and common sense. In other words, it must possess both *nursing, scientific, commonsense* and *philosophical credibility*. A theory that ignores the concerns of nursing (such as holistic care) contradicts the conclusions of science and our commonsense views about the world and fails to stand up to appropriate standards of philosophical inquiry, coherence and consistency would be unacceptable. Such a theory would also serve to perpetuate a theory–practice gap at the heart of nurse education (Timpson, 1996). It is, therefore, necessary to begin by considering what these four theoretical requirements might involve.

Nursing credibility includes elements that, to some extent like the demands of science and philosophy, evolve over time. Increasingly, allowing scope for holistic practice is considered important. This is generally said to involve four dimensions of care: biophysical, psychological, social and spiritual (although it could be argued that even such separation into dimensions undermines holism's central emphasis on unity (Goddard, 1995). The spiritual dimension is clearly important in this context, although there appears to be a lack of agreement over its meaning and role in holistic nursing (Oldnall, 1996). This holistic emphasis also represents a shift towards humanism in nursing, that is, to a reflective, person-centred approach founded on shared human experience (Playle, 1995). Consistency with nursing research values and methodology is also important. Furthermore, with regard to the consideration of nursing as a profession, it could be argued that providing a unique nursing knowledge base is also of key importance (Rose and Parker, 1994). While this should not raise barriers to coherence with other disciplines, it is clearly vital for such a theory to have unique relevance to nursing practice. Finally, a theory of mind for nursing practice should acknowledge the traditional aspects of nursing as art and science and provide a focus for the clarification and integration of this polarity.

Scientific credibility, like nursing credibility, is difficult to set out precisely, and both continue to provide scope for disagreement and debate (Playle, 1995; Paley 1996). It appears to demand coherence both with our commonsense view of the world and with the current direction of scientific research (if that is possible), in order both for nursing to be credible in practice and for nursing research to work with the findings of medicine and make use of new technology. A scientific approach (however that might be defined; see below) would also demand that a theory of mind provide a good explanation of 'the mental' (the realm of mental phenomena) and provide a basis for its study. It should also be consistent with our current best explanations of the world, such as biological evolution, while acknowledging that the aim is to be compatible with future developments in scientific inquiry rather than being tied to what we know now, especially as quantum physics is currently displacing previous scientific orthodoxy. Scientific credibility could be seen to conflict with nursing credibility in that the latter's emphasis on spirituality and holistic care, seeking to understand patients' subjective (first-person) feelings and extensive use of qualitative research methods, does not fit well with the traditional objective (third-person) and quantitative priorities of the former.

Commonsense credibility is of vital importance, especially in philosophy, since the more theoretical 'progress' is made in the debate, the more relatively obvious points tend to be disregarded or wished away. Such points include that minds cause effects in the world (your decision to pick up this book caused you to do so), that the vast majority of people you will come across today are conscious, that damage to the brain can cause mental impairment, that being shot in the leg or losing a friend feels agonisingly painful (and that such feelings really exist) and that an individual's subjective view of the world can be real and valid. Common sense can seem to conflict with scientific credibility (consider your own impression of this book, as opposed to an elemental, molecular or subatomic description of it), but to have plausibility, a theory of mind needs to reconcile these requirements.

Finally, a theory of mind needs to have philosophical credibility, which, at a general level, requires that the theory should be coherent and consistent, and should not contradict itself or collapse into a different position altogether. It would be, for example, unacceptable if the theory held that the mind both was and was not physical, or if it postulated the existence of little green men to explain itself whenever it got into difficulties. Part of the development of philosophical theories also involves finding ways of having the advantages of a position while at the same time avoiding any disadvantages. For example, if separating mind and body is seen as an advantage, this leaves the problem of how the two come to interact, while if mind and body are both physical, it is then difficult to explain how consciousness works or how mental causation takes place. Thus, philosophers may decide to abandon a theory that initially seems plausible because it turns out to lead to some unacceptable conclusions. Again, philosophical theories can wilfully disregard common sense. They may follow the lead of science and claim that we should not expect reality to conform to our perceptions of it. Such an approach is exemplified in theories of mind that seek to eliminate the mental completely or reduce it to something completely different. This is not to say that interesting arguments have not been advanced for these theories, but merely that their common-sense appeal is not particularly high.

NURSING AND THE MIND–BODY PROBLEM

The main reason for setting out the demands of nursing, scientific, commonsense and philosophical credibility at this early stage is so that the scope of the search for a theory of mind for nursing should not be underestimated. There has been a tendency in recent years for nursing theorists to attempt to give some credibility to their positions simply by linking them with bits of philosophy or other disciplines without concerning themselves with the context or applicability (or even sense) of the ideas extracted. This 'magpie' approach does nothing to enhance the professional credibility of nursing or the establishment of conceptual foundations, since little or no attention is paid to the intricacy of the issues (Paley, 1996). The main consideration when evaluating a theoretical foundation for a practice discipline such as nursing is whether or not it works for nursing and what difference it makes in practice. This is why it is necessary to keep in mind a range of examples (and counterexamples) from nursing practice when considering the theory.

The traditional mind–body problem in philosophy is perhaps best expressed by a set of questions (Nagel, 1987): what exactly *is* your mind and how is it related to your body?; does your mind inhabit your body like a ghost in a machine or is it just part of your body – your brain?; what makes you a person?, would you still be one if you had no body?; could the central features of your mind, such as consciousness, rationality and self-awareness, be purely physical?; could technology be developed which would allow others to have access to your feelings and experience your pains?; how do your mental states (your thoughts about others, your beliefs about the future, your desire to help your patients) cause physical consequences in the world? We tend to see the body as a physical thing, out in the world where everyone can see it, whereas our minds are internal and their contents private to us. Also, minds seem very unlike the purely physical things around us, such as books and bricks. Thus, it would seem that the mind has features that cannot be physical, but at the same time has strong links with the brain, which is physical. Hence, the problem is that we have reason to believe that the mind both cannot be, and is exclusively, physical (Campbell, 1984).

Is this merely another example of the unnecessary intellectualisation of a practice-based discipline? What possible relevance can this issue have to practising nurses? There are, in fact, many nursing contexts in which questions about the relation of mind to body bear on practice, perhaps the most obvious example being mental health nursing. The fact that drugs can alleviate depression shows that changes in the body and brain can affect the mind, which suggests that the mind is physical. However, the success of psychotherapy or spiritual care in a particular case might suggest that the mind is neither physical nor treatable like a burn or wound. Similarly, it could be argued that cancer patients with a fighting attitude of mind respond better to treatment, which might suggest that minds are independent of but can affect the body (Morton, 1996). A significant area of nursing expertise is in pain assessment, for example, in the case of young children, but on what basis can the nurse meet patients' needs without access to their mental states? Assumptions about pain behaviour in such contexts presuppose a view on the relation between mind and body. Altered body image (Price, 1990) and dementia (Jenkins and Price, 1996) are also relevant, in that advancing dementia may involve a transition to purely physical care at some stage, affecting the degree to which the individual is conceived of as a person, while patients' own conceptions of their bodies affect their mental well-being. Such issues illustrate the problems of separating mind and body as well as making assumptions about their integration.

Traditionally, both nursing and medicine have distinguished between mental and physical illness, under headings such as psychiatry and mental health nursing, and emphasised the importance of different skills and training in the treatment of mental and physical conditions. This would suggest, rightly or wrongly, that it is possible to treat mental health problems effectively in isolation from any concurrent physical problems and vice versa, which ties in very well with specialism in health care. In this view, people inhabit their bodies as they inhabit their cars, and if there is a problem with their tyres or they have an accident, they go and see the appropriate specialist. This does not, however, fit in with contemporary perspectives on *holism*. As Johns (1994, pp. 24–5) puts it:

> The core assumption of holism is the recognition that patients are whole people and cannot be viewed in reductionist terms, that is, as parts, systems or mind–body split... The concept of holism moves nurses away from seeing the patient within the previously dominant medical model perspective.

From a holistic perspective, individuals must be seen to have both mental and physical aspects, and, while clinical techniques may be appropriate in certain cases, health care consists of much more than this (Seedhouse and Cribb, 1989). Holistic nursing thus involves acknowledging the broader context in which individuals live, regarding them as more than the sum of their parts and also taking seriously the way people feel about their own lives – the meaning they give to them and their conceptions of uniqueness and of self. The holistic approach thus stresses the significance of subjectivity over the traditional methods of scientific objectivity. Clearly, therefore, the demands of nursing credibility, understood as placing emphasis on holistic practice, can already be seen to be opposed to the traditional distinction between mind and body. The origins of such a distinction can now be examined and subsequent developments within the philosophy of mind and nursing theory outlined.

As noted, the philosophy of mind is a wide-ranging area, incorporating many different theoretical positions. Such an area presents certain problems, such as the scope for differences of interpretation or the problem of distinguishing genuine theoretical difficulties from the sheer complexity of a theory itself. This is not to suggest that such study is either misguided or unrewarding, but it does mean that a detailed motivation and discussion of even the most relevant parts of the field is unfortunately beyond the scope of this short chapter. While it can be rather irritating constantly to be directed away to other sources, it will be necessary to refer the reader to a range of other works for the background and theoretical detail that cannot be provided here (see Guttenplan, 1994; Warner and Szubka, 1994). For now, we move on to consider, first dualism in the philosophy of mind, and then materialism.

DUALISM

Accepting that bodies are physical, extended in space, can be divided up into parts and are publicly observable, while minds are spiritual, not extended in space, indivisible and inaccessible to others, might suggest that minds and bodies are completely different kinds of thing altogether. The view that there are non-physical minds as well as physical objects in the world is known as (substance) *dualism*, and is associated with the 17th-century philosopher, Descartes (hence Cartesian dualism). Such a view might seem plausible owing to religious convictions about the immortality of the soul or from the way in which the mind appears through introspection. Descartes himself attempted to prove conclusively that mind and body are distinct. In the context of nursing, the beneficial effects of counselling on a patient's recovery, or a patient's need to find spiritual meaning in suffering, as well as the recognition of the importance of holistic care, all seem to point to the existence of a dimension to people which cannot be explained purely in physical terms, all of which might be said to give dualism some commonsense credibility.

Holden (1991) defends Cartesian dualism as a theory of mind and body for nursing practice. She argues that dualism is the only theory capable of acknowledging the mental and spiritual aspects of holistic care, termed the art of nursing, as well as the technological aspects of nursing as science. Thus, dualism is claimed to have both nursing credibility and scientific credibility. Rejection of dualism, claims Holden, leaves only two options for nursing. These are *idealism*, which is (basically) the theory that only minds exist or that everything is mental and which Holden plausibly rejects as having no commonsense or scientific credibility, and *materialism*, which is (in outline) the theory that everything is physical, and which Holden regards as having no nursing credibility. Holden asserts that, faced with this choice, the problems associated with dualism 'pale into insignificance' (Holden, 1991, p. 1377). Unfortunately, this is not the case, since dualism has no philosophical credibility whatsoever.

The main problem for any theory separating the mental and the physical is to demonstrate how they interact, as they obviously do in human beings. However, if it is suggested that this takes place in the brain, for example, the brain would have to be both mental and physical; yet, according to (substance) dualism, it can only be one or the other. Descartes himself conspicuously failed to show convincingly how interaction is possible. Also, spiritual substance remains elusive and provides no explanatory advantages in treating mental illness, for example. Similarly, dualism fails to reflect what we already know about the links between the mind and brain (the so-called neural dependence of mental phenomena). As Churchland (1988) points out, the qualified success of drugs that affect the chemistry of the brain in controlling mental illness, as well as the effects of brain damage on mental capability, both suggest strong links between mind and brain, which we would not expect were the mind a *substance entirely different* from the brain. Furthermore, evolutionary theory suggests that human beings are the result of a purely physical process going back to much simpler organisms showing no signs of mental life. Thus, it is very difficult to see how and when non-physical minds make their appearance, over and above the problem of how any particular non-spatial, non-extended mind is matched with a particular spatially extended body, all of which should provide sufficient reason to conclude with McGinn (1982, p. 25), as follows:

The objections to dualism... have not always been found decisive, and there are ways – more or less ad hoc – of clinging to the doctrine in the face of them. But dualism is evidently an extravagant and metaphysically repellent theory – a theory we would do better to improve upon if we could.

MATERIALISM AND SCIENTIFIC CREDIBILITY

Improvements on dualism have tended to involve versions of *materialism* or (more recently) versions of *physicalism* or *naturalism*, which rest on the premise, agreeable to contemporary common sense, that everything is, at least in principle, completely describable and explainable in terms of the physical (natural) sciences. This thesis, known also as the *explanatory adequacy of physics*, thus implies that the mental is physical (Warner and Szubka, 1994). In practice, this translates as a confidence in the explanatory power of science to explain the mental (mental illness becomes simply a variety of physical illness) and thus incurs great scientific credibility. By explaining away minds, spirit and mental substance, these theories avoid the problem of interaction and reflect the idea that mind depends on brain but disagree about the nature of this dependence.

At one end of the spectrum, the *mind–brain identity theory* reduces mind to brain, while, at the other end, *eliminativism* seeks to eliminate the mental completely (see Churchland, 1988); there are many different theories in between (Guttenplan, 1994). Also, materialisms exemplify a whole range of scientific virtues, such as explanatory success (in psychiatry and neurology, for example), simplicity and unity in positing only one substance, as well as the removal of folklore and superstition. Thus, pinning down the mental and understanding it for what it is need not constitute 'a gloom in which our inner life is eclipsed or suppressed, but rather a dawning' (Churchland, 1988, p. 179) in which better understanding could pave the way for genuinely holistic care. Furthermore, Holden (1991, p. 1379) cites a view according to which the central pillar of holism is unification that 'can consist of a complex of interacting parts that are both interrelated and interdependent and form a unique totality'. This would appear (despite Holden's view to the contrary) to be eminently compatible with the unity provided by a one-substance materialism!

However, neither elimination nor reduction seems able to account for certain important features of the mental and thus lose nursing, commonsense and philosophical credibility. Both fail to do justice to the mind as revealed by introspection, its inner qualities and subjectivity. A good example of this is altered body image. How is it possible to help patients who have suffered a major physical change to their body to recover without taking account of their own subjective feelings about it? This is not to say that introspection necessarily reveals things as they really are but merely that what science has to say about something is not necessarily all there is to say about it (Guttenplan, 1994). The complexities of consciousness are not reflected in these theories, nor are the felt qualities (sometimes referred to as qualia) of mental states. Pain, for example, may be felt as burning, jabbing or throbbing. Assessment of pain, as in young children, for example, will depend on patients' own feelings as much as on data received from monitoring their physical states. This objection could be captured in the suggestion that knowing facts about someone's brain (and body) does not allow one to know what it is like to be that person (Morton, 1996).

Attempts have been made to come up with improved versions of materialism, such as *anomalous monism* and *functionalism*. Although well worth exploring, discussion of these developments is beyond the scope of this paper. It worth noting, in passing, that, in spite of their having many advantages over standard versions, these theories still appear to fall victim to one or more of the problems that face materialisms generally. Such problems include omitting to take the phenomenon of consciousness seriously, failure to give the mind sufficient causal power over physical effects and failure to explain the directedness (so-called *intentionality*) of mental attitudes (thoughts, beliefs and desires about the world). There are, of course, those who would dispute the above verdict on these theories, and readers are strongly encouraged to review the original sources and make up their own minds on these theories of mind. (On *anomalous monism*, see Davidson, 1980; on *functionalism*, see Guttenplan, 1994.)

Further problems for materialism arise from contemporary views of nursing. Nursing as an art is characterised for Holden by 'the caring role' (1991, p. 1375), while nursing as science is associated with 'high technology'. A theory of mind that regards mind and body as fundamentally the same, single thing provides grounds for nursing as a *science*, but, argues Holden, it is not adequate to ground the psychological and spiritual aspects of nursing practice, seen as an art. Johns (1994, p. 9) also has doubts about the scope for holistic practice of such a theory and the problems for nursing caused by a reductionist approach, in which things are explained by breaking them down into their physical components:

> I have a deep uneasiness about nursing if it requires nursing models to tell human-beings (nurses) that other human-beings (patients and their families) are in reality also human-beings. This is a deeply

shocking notion that reflects how reductionist nursing practice and health care in general has become. Human-beings are clearly not objects to be taken apart.

Similarly, Oldnall (1996) argues that spirituality's refusal to be quantified easily, or researched using scientific methods, means that it is perceived as a threat to nursing's scientific credibility. Goddard (1995) blames the general adherence to materialistic monism for the neglect of the spiritual dimension and consequent undermining of holism in nursing. Holism, it would seem, is not compatible with materialism, which would appear to constitute a major obstacle to achieving both scientific and nursing credibility in the same theory.

HOLISM AND CONTINENTAL PHILOSOPHY

Benner and Wrubel (1989) share these concerns about holistic care and develop them into a different approach to the nature of persons taken from continental philosophy. Benner and Wrubel reject Cartesian dualism, insisting that 'the mind and body are not dual realities as the Cartesian tradition of a mind/body (subject/object) split portrays' (1989, p. xii). They also oppose the reductionism implied by materialism. Both dualism and materialism are regarded as obstructing a proper understanding of health and illness. Benner and Wrubel (1989, p. 22) quote Cassell (1982, p. 640) on the problems this creates:

> Where the mind is problematic (not identifiable in objective terms), its reality diminishes for science, and so, too, does that of the person. Therefore, so long as the mind–body dichotomy is accepted, suffering is either subjective and not truly 'real' – not within medicine's domain – or identified exclusively with bodily pain.

Furthermore, the Cartesian view is claimed to lead to a position in which human subjects are regarded as objects for the purposes of scientific explanation, with the result that the person 'cannot be seen as a creative, generating being who lives embedded in a context of meaning, a being whose actions and understandings form a comprehensible whole' (Benner and Wrubel, 1989, p. 35).

Benner and Wrubel follow Heidegger (1962) in rejecting the distinction between subject and object, which is traced back to Descartes, in favour of a view, which seeks to unify mind and body into a concept of a person who is seen as embodied and participating in a meaningful world. While the Cartesian view identifies the self with a rational mind that is separated from everything else, Heidegger stresses the importance of context as a basis for understanding the self in the world, regarding the person as a self-interpreting being and as involved in a situation, rather than standing outside it, all of which provides a sound basis for a profound understanding of holistic care. (See Leonard, 1989, for an excellent summary of Heidegger's notoriously difficult views.)

What of the credibility of Benner and Wrubel's approach to the issues? Holden (1991) accuses them of failing to refute dualism and adhering to idealism. The former charge, if correct, has been answered above, and the latter is not clear. The term 'idealism' in philosophy has many different senses and uses (Dawson, 1994), and it is not clear that a Heideggerian approach is by definition idealist (in the worst sense) simply because it rejects dualism, so these objections are not serious. Benner and Wrubel also avoid Holden's challenge that holism is incompatible with materialism by rejecting materialism and thus retaining nursing credibility with the scope for holistic care. Regarding philosophical credibility, it is important to bear in mind the nature of the differences, both in approach and in attitude, between analytic and continental philosophy. Heideggerian philosophy differs radically from Anglo-American approaches, although this is not to imply that it has no philosophical credibility (depending on how this is assessed).

Benner and Wrubel do not identify any problems for their view, although viewing 'the body itself [as] a knower and interpreter' might stretch commonsense credibility somewhat (1989, p. 409). However, there would appear to be a significant problem of scientific credibility. In rejecting the distinction between subject and object and between knower and known, Heidegger removes the ground from under the entire scientific enterprise, and it is not clear what methods of research could then be used. The problem is that Heidegger's philosophy is not some optional extra, which can be combined with other theoretical components, but an entirely different world-view (Dreyfus, 1991). While such a world-view might provide exactly the foundation that nursing requires, it might also lead to conceptual problems and demand sacrifices that nursing is unable, or unwilling, to make.

CHALLENGING CURRENT ORTHODOXY: EMERGENTIST MATERIALISM

While continental philosophy might seem a promising route for nursing, Dawson (1994) has argued in favour of occupying the middle ground of compromise rather than pledging undying allegiance to any one particular theory. Dawson contests Holden's (1991) view of Cartesian dualism and argues that Benner and Wrubel's concept of 'wholeness' is in fact perfectly compatible with a materialist emphasis, thus rejecting Holden's challenge. He also rejects the tendency within nursing (Holden, 1991) to identify the mental with nursing as art and the physical with nursing as science. Furthermore, he stresses the need for 'a metatheory which would integrate the functioning of the mental and physical realms, and dissolve the somewhat arbitrary distinction between art and science' (Dawson, 1994, p. 1017).

Dawson (1994) seeks such integration in what he refers to as *emergentist materialism*, which allows for emergent entities and attributes that cannot be characterised solely in physical terms and stresses the importance of personhood, with its cultural and social emphasis, and embodiment (Benner and Wrubel, 1989), claiming that this version of materialism avoids the problems of dualism and provides nursing credibility through holistic care. Thus, Dawson demonstrates how it is possible, in principle at least, to explore links and compromise (including between analytic and continental traditions) in constructing a theory, rather than focusing on extremes, but he also questions the need for a theory of mind at all, encouraging flexibility rather than the championing of one viewpoint to the exclusion of all others.

Dawson also considers that traditional materialist science, as conceived by Holden (1991) (see above), is unhelpful for nursing and that the view of science as objective is an outdated one, arguing that contemporary quantum theory exhibits properties of wholeness and connectedness, which traditional Newtonian physics does not. This view is shared by Paley (1996), who stresses the need for nursing theorists to bring their conception of science up to date by incorporating recent developments. However, rather than insisting that the notion of scientific credibility be re-evaluated on this basis, Dawson questions the need for a theory of mind to revolve around scientific method at all, on the basis that science is itself a cultural, rather than an objective and value-free, enterprise. Moreover, he applauds nursing's focus on holistic care as leading the way against the traditional and increasingly discredited reductionist and materialist approaches. Playle (1995) also identifies unhelpful polarisation and conflict between the holistic conception of nursing as art and the positivist, traditionally scientific, conception of nursing as science and calls for a re-definition of nursing science that 'acknowledges the importance of subjective experience and... the centrality of the personal' (1995, p. 983). Dawson's proposal for an approach to the mind would seem to provide a basis for such a re-definition.

However, while there is much to be learned from Dawson's argument, it is not clear that an approach based on emergentist materialism is unquestionably the way to go. Emergence, like idealism, is variously interpreted, but the suggestion that mental properties somehow come about once purely physical systems have evolved sufficient complexity does not combine well with a simultaneous *rejection* of their reduction to the physical components from which they emerged (Churchland, 1988). Others regard emergentism as too much like accepting miracles or simply positing a mystery to explain a mystery – a tactic with little scientific, commonsense or philosophical credibility (McGinn, 1994).

As Warner (1994) stresses, a helpful question to consider (especially with respect to patients in the context of scientific credibility and the character of mental life) is 'Am I an object fully describable and explainable by science?' While the prevailing answer, reflecting traditional scientific credibility would be 'Yes', Benner and Wrubel and Dawson take a different view, and there are other dissenters within analytic philosophy. Pessimistically, Nagel (1994) argues that an acceptable theory of consciousness that takes subjectivity seriously would have to be fundamentally different from current theory and could not be generated by current methods of explanation. McGinn (1994) goes further, suggesting that consciousness is, in principle, inexplicable because our concepts are inadequate to capture it. More optimistically, Searle (1992) argues in favour of a return to common sense about the mind while challenging the hold of traditional scientific credibility in a way which provides a more promising foundation for a theory of mind for nursing.

BREAKING THE HOLD: BIOLOGICAL NATURALISM

Searle (1992) helps to clarify the philosophical credibility that any theory of mind must possess by returning to the demands of common sense about the mind. He rules out reduction and elimination of the mental and sets out to show that it is possible to accept that the world is physical without denying the reality of biological phenomena such as inner, subjective qualitative states of consciousness – how it feels to be in pain, for example. This still raises many questions yet to be answered, such as the nature of consciousness, the special features of the mental and the causal relations between mental and physical.

However, most importantly, *biological naturalism* provides an alternative to dualism and materialism, the obvious falsity of which, while being regarded as the only available options, has (according to Searle) obstructed development in recent philosophy of mind.

Searle's (1992) arguments against the varieties of materialism merit serious consideration, but perhaps his most relevant point here is that not all of reality is objective. Some things, such as consciousness or feelings of pain, are *subjective*, so traditional science, with its emphasis on the third-person perspective, objectivity and publicly observable phenomena, is simply not the one and only method and source of knowledge about reality. Thus, the traditional view of scientific credibility is once again challenged. Rather than the success of scientific methods showing that consciousness and subjectivity are unreal, the existence of consciousness and subjectivity demonstrate the limits of a purely objectifying, third-person approach.

Just as Heidegger rejects the Cartesian subject–object world-view completely, Searle argues that materialism is to be rejected because it accepts the dualist starting point of the separation of the world into mental and physical categories. However, Searle (1992) cites Dreyfus (1991) as showing that even Heidegger and his followers doubt the importance of consciousness and intentionality. Searle stresses that, in order to take these obvious features of the mind seriously, it is necessary to reconsider the vocabulary of the debate and the accompanying categories, which undermine debate by structuring our thinking in rigid and unhelpful ways. Finally, unlike Nagel and McGinn, Searle does not consider that understanding the nature of consciousness is necessarily beyond us, the problem is simply that 'we cannot get at the reality of consciousness in the way that, using consciousness, we can get at the reality of other phenomena' (1992, pp. 96–7), a situation which the whole development of holistic nursing is already acknowledging.

TOWARDS A THEORY OF MIND FOR NURSING

Whatever the defects or virtues of Searle's view, it certainly opens up new directions and goes a long way towards breaking the hold of the prevailing views within philosophy of mind in recent years. However, we should note with Nagel (1979, p. 193) that 'there is no reason to think that all possibilities have been thought of, so there is no reason to assume that a view is correct if all currently conceivable alternatives are even more unacceptable'. Either way, Searle provides an opportunity to review the criteria introduced above for a credible theory of mind for nursing practice.

As Dawson (1994) points out, it is only recently that nursing has begun to reflect on practice and begun to establish philosophical foundations, but the importance of establishing *nursing credibility* is rapidly increasing. As has been shown, what works for nursing is the central criterion here. Developments in holistic care must continue to be the focus for theory development, without worrying about whether the methodology is consistent with traditional science.

Regarding *scientific credibility*, there is clearly a need to reassess what this means, both in the light of recent developments in the sciences and in view of nursing's humanistic focus for practice. However, there is no reason why a theory of mind that takes consciousness and subjectivity seriously and provides an integrated view of the person could not break down not only the mind–body distinction, but also the nursing-as-art-or-science distinction. What this discussion does show, as Dawson (1994) emphasises, is the importance of breaking down obstructive barriers, which are more often artefacts of an outdated way of thinking than genuine theoretical problems.

Integration and compromise will be inappropriate, however, where theories and views are inconsistent and contradictory, so the demands of *philosophical credibility* need to be adhered to. A theory of mind for nursing with philosophical credibility must, as has been shown, avoid reduction, elimination and outdated Cartesian intuitions about the self, take consciousness, subjectivity and intentionality seriously, allow for mental causation and the felt quality of mental states (qualia) and remain consistent with the explanatory adequacy of physics. As far as *commonsense credibility* is concerned, this is not so much to say that a theory must reflect current wisdom, since many correct theories (for example, heliocentrism) have come into conflict with contemporary thinking, but to prevent theories from flouting what we already know about the mind from our daily interactions with others. As Searle (1992) argues, the more theoretical the discussion, the easier it is to lose sight of the basic features of the mind, which once again illustrates the importance of grounding a theory of mind in nursing practice, as the provision of practice examples has sought to show.

These four areas of credibility – nursing, scientific, commonsense and philosophical – can, of course, be used to assess and construct a whole range of conceptual foundations for nursing, which should then provide a fully integrated theoretical base, able to respond to the changing needs of practice. However, while philosophy can be a useful tool in achieving this, we should note with Holden (1991, p. 1381) that 'it behoves us to treat philosophy with more respect and ensure that we have grasped the real meaning of the various philosophical positions we proselytize for mass consumption'.

ACKNOWLEDGEMENTS

The author would like to thank Steven Edwards, Trevor Hussey and Mark Fielding for helpful discussions.

REFERENCES

Benner, P. and Wrubel, J. (1989) *The Primacy of Caring* (Menlo Park, CA: Addison-Wesley).

Campbell, K. (1984) *Body and Mind*, 2nd edn (Indiana: University of Notre Dame Press).

Cassell, E.J. (1982) The nature of suffering and the goals of medicine, *New England Journal of Medicine*, **30**: 639–40.

Churchland, P. (1988) *Matter and Consciousness* (Cambridge, MA: MIT Press).

Davidson, D. (1980) *Essays on Actions and Events* (Oxford: Oxford University Press).

Dawson, P.J. (1994) In defence of the middle ground, *Journal of Advanced Nursing* **19**: 1015–23.

Descartes, R. (1994) *Meditations on First Philosophy and Discourse on the Method* (London: Everyman).

Dreyfus, H. (1991) *Being-in-the-world: A Commentary on Heidegger's Being and Time: Division I* (Cambridge, MA: MIT Press).

Goddard, N.C. (1995) Spirituality as integrative energy: a philosophical analysis as requisite precursor to holistic nursing practice, *Journal of Advanced Nursing*, **22**: 808–15.

Guttenplan, S. (ed.) (1994) *A Companion to the Philosophy of Mind* (Oxford: Blackwell).

Haldane, J.J. (1994) Analytical philosophy and the nature of mind: time for another rebirth?, in Warner, R. and Szubka, T. (eds) *The Mind–Body Problem: A Guide to the Current Debate*, pp. 195–203 (Oxford: Blackwell).

Heidegger, M. (1962, trans. J. Macquarrie and E. Robinson) *Being and Time*, (New York: Harper & Row).

Holden, R.J. (1991) In defence of Cartesian dualism and the hermeneutic horizon, *Journal of Advanced Nursing*, **16**: 1375–81.

Jenkins, D. and Price, R. (1996) Dementia and personhood: a focus for care?, *Journal of Advanced Nursing*, **24** : 84–90.

Johns, C. (ed.) (1994) *The Burford NDU Model: Caring in Practice* (Oxford: Blackwell Science).

Johnson, J.L. (1994) A dialectical examination of nursing art, *Advances in Nursing Science*, **17**(1): 1–14.

Kim, J. (1994) The myth of non-reductive materialism, in Warner, R. and Szubka, T. (eds) *The Mind–Body Problem: A Guide to the Current Debate*, pp. 242–60 (Oxford: Blackwell).

Kramer, M.K. (1990) Holistic nursing: implications for knowledge development and utilization in Chaska, N.L, (ed.) *The Profession of Nursing*, (St, Louis: C.V. Mosby).

Leonard, V.W. (1989) A Heideggerian phenomenological perspective on the concept of person, *Advances in Nursing Science*, **11**: 40–55.

Macdonald, C. (1989) *Mind–Body Identity Theories* (London: Routledge).

McGinn, C. (1982) *The Character of Mind* (Oxford: Oxford University Press).

McGinn, C. (1994) Can we solve the mind–body problem?, in Warner, R. and Szubka, T. (eds) *The Mind–Body Problem: A Guide to the Current Debate*, pp. 99–120 (Oxford: Blackwell).

Morton, A. (1996) *Philosophy in Practice* (Oxford: Blackwell).

Nagel, T. (1979) Panpsychism, in Nagel, T. *Mortal Questions*, pp. 181–95 (Cambridge: Cambridge University Press).

Nagel, T. (1987) *What Does It All Mean? A Very Short Introduction to Philosophy* (New York: Oxford University Press).

Nagel, T. (1994) 'Consciousness and objective reality', in Warner, R. and Szubka, T. (eds) *The Mind–Body Problem: A Guide to the Current Debate*, pp. 63–78 (Oxford: Blackwell).

Oldnall, A. (1996) A critical analysis of nursing: meeting the spiritual needs of patients, *Journal of Advanced Nursing*, **23**: 138–44.

Paley, J. (1996) Intuition and expertise: comments on the Benner debate, *Journal of Advanced Nursing*, **23**: 665–71.

Paterson, J.G. and Zderad, L.T. (eds) (1976) *Humanistic Nursing* (New York: John Wiley).

Playle, J.F. (1995) Humanism and positivism in nursing: contradictions and conflicts, *Journal of Advanced Nursing*, **22**: 979–84.

Price, B. (1990) *Body Image: Nursing Concepts and Care* (Hemel Hempstead: Prentice-Hall International).

Rose, P. and Parker, D. (1994) Nursing: an integration of art and science within the experience of the practitioner, *Journal of Advanced Nursing*, **20**: 1004–10.

Searle, J.R. (1992) *The Rediscovery of the Mind* (Cambridge, MA: MIT Press).

Seedhouse, D. and Cribb, A. (eds) (1989) *Changing Ideas in Health Care* (Chichester: John Wiley).

Timpson, J. (1996) Nursing theory: everything the artist spits is art?, *Journal of Advanced Nursing*, **23**:1030–6.

Warner, R. (1994) Introduction: the mind–body debate, in Warner, R. and Szubka, T. (eds) *The Mind–Body Problem: A Guide to the Current Debate*, pp. 1–16 (Oxford: Blackwell).

Warner, R. and Szubka, T. (eds) (1994) *The Mind–Body Problem: A Guide to the Current Debate* (Oxford: Blackwell).

Part III

The Nurse Curriculum

CHAPTER SEVEN

Heidegger and the
nurse curriculum

EDITOR'S INTRODUCTION

In this chapter, Stephen Horrocks shows how the philosophical programme of Heidegger has application to the nursing context, specifically, to nurse education. Horrocks suggests that Cartesian conceptions of mind have helped to foster the presumption that theoretical knowledge precedes, or is more fundamental than, practical knowledge ('know-how').

Horrocks recruits Heidegger's distinction between that which is 'present-at-hand' and that which is 'ready-to-hand' (roughly, the distinction between the theoretical and practical perspectives). Following Heidegger, Horrocks argues that theoretical knowledge must be grounded in practice. Hence, models of nurse education that begin with theory, in the expectation that nurses will apply this in practice, are seriously flawed. The place to learn is the world of practice.

Moreover, as Horrocks indicates, it is not at all clear that much of the knowledge necessary for practice can be acquired or taught in the classroom as such knowledge is not reducible to step-by-step sequences of instructions. The acquisition of knowledge necessary for nursing practice requires immersement into the world of practice. It is in this world that the student learns to make the fine discriminations and judgements necessary for competent practice; this is a mode of awareness termed 'circumspection' by Heidegger, and this too can only be acquired in the practical context.

Heidegger and the nurse curriculum

Stephen Horrocks

Much good work has been written regarding the application of the philosophy of Heidegger (1889–1976) to the nursing context. However, a good deal of this has centred on Benner's (1984) concept of intuition and has ignored the wider context of Heidegger's thought, specifically, that which concerns an 'ontological shift' from 'theoretical thinking' to 'practical thinking' (in Heidegger's terminology, from the present-at-hand to the ready-to-hand). Crudely, Heidegger's proposal is that the relationship between theory and practice has been mistakenly inverted. We take it to be the case that it is theoretical knowledge which is considered most important. However, Heidegger claims that this is not the case, first, owing to the fact that theory arises out of practice and hence is parasitic upon it, and second, owing to the fact that theory must not be divorced from practice.

In Heidegger's terms, the ready-to-hand (the world of practice) provides the 'ground' of the present-at-hand (the world of theory). Given that this is the case, it may be possible to derive theory from consideration of practice, but it is not possible to derive theory independently of consideration of practice. So, again crudely, Heidegger seeks to show that theoretical knowledge (knowledge of that which is present-at-hand) is grounded in practical knowledge (knowledge of the ready-to-hand). What I therefore intend to do in this paper is to look closely at the above-mentioned 'ontological shift' and the implications it has for the nurse curriculum.

HEIDEGGER AND HUSSERL

In order properly to understand the relevance of Heidegger's work to nurse education, it is necessary to contrast his form of phenomenology with that of Husserl (1859–1938). Husserl attempted to describe his own mental experiences and, by focusing exclusively and painstakingly on these, to discover all that we can know about the world. Roughly speaking, Husserl's project is conducted from that of the first-person perspective, and it is supposed that the integrity of this perspective owes nothing to phenomena beyond it, that is, to objects outside the minds of persons.

It is this introspective, or first-person, focus that Heidegger challenges. Husserl is charged with adopting a Cartesian starting point – a point from which the sole thing a person can be certain of is his own existence. This starting point presumes a 'gap' or separation between the person (the thinking subject) and the world that he occupies. Once posited, this gap becomes increasingly difficult to bridge, and the question of how contact is possible between the thinking subject and independently existing objects remains an insoluble problem.

Husserl attempted to re-connect the subject with the world (in essence, to bridge the gap) by positing 'intentional contents'. Basically, these are representations, or mental images, of things in the world. Phenomenology, in the Husserlian account, then consists in the study of these intentional contents (thoughts, mental images, representations and so on). He thus defined phenomenology as the study of the intentional content (thoughts and so on) remaining in the mind after the world has been, so to speak, 'bracketed off'.

To gain access to this mental content in consciousness, Husserl posited a special type of reflection, a type of reflection:

> in which we turn our attention *away from* the object being referred to (and *away from* our psychological experience of being directed toward that object), and turn our attention to the act, more specifically to its intentional content, thus making our representation of the conditions of satisfaction of the intentional state our object. (Dreyfus, 1984, p. 6)

Thus, Husserl's focus of enquiry lies with that which remains 'inside' consciousness – what was described earlier as intentional content (that is, representations of 'external objects', ideas, thoughts and mental images).

Heidegger objected to Husserl's insistence that all objects be treated as intentional objects, that is, as objects represented in consciousness. It is this notion, that of 'representations in consciousness', which is the crucial point of difference between Heidegger and Husserl. Put simply, in a Husserlian account of the relationship between persons and the world they occupy, the person has mental representations of things in the world. As noted, this suggests that the relationship between the person and the world is a detached one: the person and his mental representations are separable from the world inhabited by the person. However, for Heidegger, the very idea of such a separation is misconceived. For him, persons are not separable from the world they inhabit. Nor, for Heidegger, is it legitimate to claim that persons have mental representations that are independent of items in the world.

So the crucial point of difference between the two philosophers may be put thus. Husserl's project presumes that persons and their mental states are separable from the contexts that they inhabit. Heidegger's project is fundamentally opposed to the very idea of such a separation. Heidegger in this way sought to shift the focus of phenomenology away from consciousness and into the everydayness of 'lived experience'. This, he suggests, is where the understanding of all intentionality, or thought, must be grounded.

In terms of the theory/practice distinction referred to at the start of this paper, Heidegger's focus on 'lived experience' is supposed to uncover just what it is that makes the kind of theoretical thinking about the relationship between the thinking human subject and the world she inhabits possible. His claim is that such theoretical thinking cannot legitimately be shorn from the world of everyday experience. It is this latter which makes theoretical thinking possible.

It is important to emphasise that Heidegger's starting point is not self-consciousness, nor the information available from the first-person perspective on thought but rather what makes such a theoretical orientation possible. In other words, Heidegger is seeking to discover a phenomenology that underpins Husserl's, that is presupposed by Husserl's project and is thus more fundamental.

THEORY AND PRACTICE

Heidegger identifies two ways in which humans relate to the things that surround them. The first is a theoretical way of thinking about things, which he terms the 'present-at-hand' stance. Another way of relating to objects is found in the way in which humans simply use them: think of tools, utensils and so on. This mode of relating to things is termed by Heidegger the 'ready-to-hand' stance. Heidegger argues that the present-at-hand stance treats all knowledge as theoretical and is epistemological. However, as noted, there is, he supposes, another way in which humans relate to objects, such as that which takes place in the practical world of the ready-to-hand.

It can be pointed out that this latter ready-to-hand world does not involve intentional content at all. That is to say, in our dealings with objects at a practical level, it does not seem to be the case that our actions are informed by mental representations of such objects or by following mental images of step-by-step instructions. In activities such as driving, typing or eating, we simply perform these without any resort to 'inner' mental representations.

It should be stressed that Heidegger is not claiming that mental states derive their intentional content via a connection with the external world. Heidegger wants to reject completely the notion of a mental content that is 'purely' mental. For Heidegger, there is a way of relating to the world that involves no mediation between mental content and the world. This aspect of Heidegger's work deeply influenced Benner's concept of 'intuition' as it is described in her *From Novice to Expert* (1984). It also has major ramifications for the way in which the relationship between theory and practice is understood, for, if Heidegger is correct, there is no 'pure' theory underlying practice.

So Heidegger's claims, if applied to the context of nurse education, or indeed to the educative aspect of any practice-based activity, could be very important indeed. They imply that practice and the experience of practice are absolutely essential components of any educative programme. Furthermore, they suggest that it is the practical rather than the theoretical components of education which are the most crucial.

Heidegger's use of the term 'world'

Traditional philosophical approaches to the problem of knowledge (the problem of what knowledge is) typically proceed by aiming to conduct objective, detached inquiry. This involves stepping back from our ordinary, everyday experiences of situations and coolly reflecting upon them. However, in doing this, it could be asked whether one is in fact moving away from the real source of knowledge and understanding of our experience. For, in moving further away from everyday practice, we would appear to be moving away from the source of knowledge and understanding of everyday practices.

Consider an experienced nurse who, following a day's work, reflects upon a practical situation that he encountered during the day. Does such a nurse import theories into his understanding of the situation or does he use his vast amount of practical experience to help make sense of the situation? In order to answer this question, it is necessary to look at what Heidegger means by the term 'world' as it figures in Heidegger's technical term 'Being-in-the-world'. (Roughly speaking, the term 'Being-in-the-world' refers to an holistic concept; it is hyphenated to denote that the terms 'Being' and 'world' are inseparable.)

For Heidegger, standard philosophical attempts to understand the nature of the world interpret the term 'world' as the world of the theoretical present-at-hand. Thus, as in Husserl, the world is seen as separable from the human subject or, to use Heidegger's term for individual human beings, 'Dasein'. However, if 'world' is interpreted as a state of Dasein in its everydayness – that is, as not separable from the human subject – what is closest to Dasein is its *environment* (Heidegger, 1980, p. 94), that is, the context that an individual person inhabits. This context, of course, is typically a social one including inanimate objects, persons and so on. It comprises those entities which we encounter as closest to us within the environment of Being-in-the-world.

Heidegger describes our interactions with these objects, as our *dealings in* with the world. He explains the notion of 'dealing' as follows:

> The kind of dealing which is closest to us is as we have shown, not a bare perceptual cognition, but rather that kind of concern which manipulates things and puts them to use; and this has its own kind of 'knowledge'. (1980, p. 95)

In other words, there is no representation of the environment of the practical ready-to-hand 'world' as there is for the theoretical, present-at-hand 'world'. If the environment of the ready-to-hand 'world' is known in a way unique to it, it will be a type of knowledge distinct from that which is recruited in understanding of the present-at-hand 'world'. The kind of knowledge relevant to the practical world is that involved in knowing how to do things and how to manipulate objects, pieces of equipment and so on. It is evident that our standard dealings with such items do not involve mental representations of them. Typically, we simply perform the relevant acts without any conscious reflection. The items or entities that occupy the practical world:

> are not thereby objects for knowing the 'world' theoretically; they are simply what gets used, what gets produced, and so forth. (Heidegger, 1980, p. 95).

A closer examination of this type of ready-to-hand knowledge should reveal how this knowledge is acquired. Bear in mind that it is a type of knowledge which we do not have to think about and which is situated in the 'world'.

So far then, we have noted that there is, for Heidegger, the world of the present-at-hand and the world of the ready-to-hand. The world of the ready-to-hand is not separable from a context or local environment, and this environment is composed of objects that stand in various relations to each other. An important feature of some of these objects, especially in the world of practice, is that they are items of equipment.

'Equipment'

Heidegger describes certain of the entities that we encounter in our environment as 'equipment', giving examples such as doorknobs and latches. In the nursing context, we might identify sphygmomanometers and thermometers. Heidegger goes on to suggest that there is no such thing as *an* equipment. Equipment is inevitably related to other items of equipment. Equipment belongs to a totality of equipment. It is always 'something in-order-to'; in other words, it has a use, and, as noted, it is related to other items of equipment.

Heidegger suggests that, when we enter a room, we encounter the room not as something spatial, in a geometric sense, but as something with equipment residing in it. These items of equipment may then become evident, individually, to the person. Furthermore, according to Heidegger, it is important to note that the totality of equipment in a room shows itself before the individual items of equipment. Thus, in entering into a room full of equipment, one does not single out an individual item but surveys a totality of equipment (think of the first time one steps onto a busy hospital ward).

For example, it can be pointed out that, typically, nurses are located in the context of the clinical environment before they seek out individual items of equipment. Moreover, the individual items of equipment in the clinical environment are not thought of in a theoretical, present-at-hand way (at least, this is true for experienced nurses in familiar circumstances). The concern of the nurse in the clinical context is focused on the 'in-order-to' or functional structure of the context or 'world'. The equipment in such contexts is said by Heidegger to be ready-to-hand, in contrast to present-at-hand; that is, the items of equipment are not thought of theoretically.

In order to appreciate more of what is involved in the nature of the relation between the person and the equipment in her environment, it is important to consider Heidegger's notion of 'circumspection'. Basically, this amounts to looking around an environment and the equipment in it, but doing so in a non-theoretical manner.

'Circumspection'

Heidegger writes:

> If we look at Things just 'theoretically', we can get along without understanding readiness-to-hand. But when we deal with them by using them and manipulating them, this activity is not a blind one; it

has its own kind of sight, by which our manipulation is guided and from which it acquires its specific Thingly character. Dealings with equipment subordinate themselves to the manifold assignments of the 'in-order-to'. And the sight with which they thus accommodate themselves is *circumspection*. (1980, p. 98)

In this passage, Heidegger asserts a special kind of 'sight' or knowledge that is involved in the way we use equipment or tools. He also indicates that 'circumspection' is an especially important element of this. Moreover, it is evident that the terms 'using' and 'manipulating' are also considered central, so a word about these terms is needed.

As we have seen, the use of equipment in the context in which it is used is in some ways more fundamental than a detached, theoretical thinking about it. Also, as noted, equipment is always located within a context of other equipment to which it is related. The basic way of understanding equipment is to 'use it'; this mode of understanding Heidegger terms 'manipulating'. However, when we are using equipment, it becomes transparent. For example:

When an expert carpenter is hammering – if the hammer is working well, and he is master at what he is doing – the hammer becomes transparent for him. He does not have to think about it at all. He might be paying attention to the nails, but if he is really good and the nails are going in well he does not have to pay attention to them either. He can think about lunch, or he can talk to some fellow carpenter, and his hammering simply goes on in a 'transparent coping' mode. (Magee, 1987, pp. 257–8)

Thus the nurse who is learning how to take blood pressure or any other practical task is better able to learn how to do this by using the relevant equipment and manipulating it. She needs to relate to the 'world' (the clinical environment) in a ready-to-hand way. If everything is going smoothly, the nurse is functioning in the 'transparent coping mode' (Magee, 1987, p. 258). As indicated in the last quotation, when we use familiar equipment it paradoxically has a tendency to 'withdraw' or 'disappear'. As Heidegger puts it:

The ready-to-hand is not grasped theoretically at all, nor is it itself the sort of thing that circumspection takes proximally as a circumspective theme. The peculiarity of what is proximally ready-to-hand is that, in its readiness-to-hand, it must, as it were, withdraw in order to be ready-to-hand quite authentically. (Heidegger, 1980, p. 99)

We make use of things, but we do not notice them when we are using them. The expert nurse who is taking the blood pressure is carrying out the procedure to get the work done; she does not need to be thinking theoretically about the physiology of blood pressure.

This suggests that any nurse in a practical situation needs to be taught the skill of 'circumspective penetration' so that she can *see* the *environment* of the 'world' around her. Consequently, if the nurse is very circumspective, the environment she is working in will become more explicit, that is, the relevant features of the clinical environment or 'world' will be evident to the nurse.

Furthermore, as noted, circumspection is said to have its own kind of sight:

> 'Practical' behaviour is not 'atheoretical' in the sense of 'sightlessness'. The way it differs from theoretical behaviour does not lie simply in the fact that in theoretical behaviour one observes, while in practical behaviour one *acts*, and that action must employ theoretical cognition if it is not to remain blind; for the fact that observation is a kind of concern is just as primordial as the fact that action has its *own* kind of sight. Theoretical behaviour is just looking, without circumspection. (Heidegger, 1980, p. 99)

Heidegger is suggesting that practical behaviour has a relationship to its environment – to the 'world' of the ready-to-hand – and that this relationship is characterised by circumspection. There is knowledge embedded in the 'world' of equipment that is different in character from that of the theoretical present-to-hand 'world'. If one is to 'think theoretically' this necessarily concerns the present-at-hand 'world' rather than the ready-to-hand 'world'. Heidegger suggests that action has its own kind of sight, which he terms circumspection. Thus, the nurse in the clinical environment needs to focus upon the world of the ready-to-hand and ignore the world of the present-at-hand.

Summary

We are now at the crux of the difficulties that surround the relationship between theory and practice. We have access to both the latter worlds – the theoretical and the practical – and we encounter both present-at-hand and ready-to-hand objects. We are now in a position to claim that nurse education needs to develop more emphasis upon the world of the ready-to-hand. The circumspection involved in looking around only makes sense in the practical background of the world of the clinical environment.

In outline, if Heidegger is right, the judgements and perceptual discriminations necessary for practice can be acquired only in the practical context. The world of the theoretical present-at-hand that has been emphasised in the nurse curriculum has been over-emphasised. Exaggeration of the role and importance of theory has led us to ignore the rich background of experience that any expert nurse brings to a practical situation. Unless one is engaged in practice first, it is difficult to take a theoretical stance, one has to be an agent rather than a spectator.

In order to prevent the nurse concerning herself with the theoretical present-at-hand world, she needs to develop the circumspection of 'looking around' the practical background of the (clinical) world. Using and manipulating equipment without the skill of circumspective penetration is blind. Of course, it might be argued that circumspection is a type of reflecting, but it is a reflecting on the practical background in which the nurse dwells and is immersed. It is not the detached reflection of Husserlian phenomenology, of the 'pure' theorist.

CIRCUMSPECTION AND THEORETICAL KNOWLEDGE

Where does one stop being circumspective and become theoretical? To answer this question, we need to consider the background, practical world much more. It must be remembered that Heidegger focuses on practical examples because they involve action, and actions seem easiest to explain without resorting to an appeal to mental representations. However, action takes place against a wider social background. The taking of blood pressure occurs within a cultural background of other shared practices. As Dreyfus suggests, these practices are typically not consciously learned but simply acquired unreflectively. He writes:

> And just as we can learn to swim without consciously or unconsciously acquiring a theory of swimming, we can acquire these social background practices by being brought up in them, not by forming beliefs and learning rules. (Dreyfus, 1980, p. 37)

What is important to note here is that the background is pervasive and the practices involve skills. From the Heideggerian perspective, the acquisition of cultural skills is not a reflective process involving mental representations. Such skills are simply absorbed through living in one's culture.

Heidegger takes great care to explore the emergence of the theoretical attitude from the practical attitude. He writes:

> In characterising the change-over from the manipulating and using and so forth which are circumspective in a 'practical' way, to 'theoretical' exploration, it would be easy to suggest that merely looking at entities is something which emerges when concern *holds back* from any kind of manipulation. What is decisive in the 'emergence' of the theoretical attitude would then lie in the *disappearance of praxis*. (Heidegger, 1980, p. 409)

Thus, if one stops being practical, the theoretical attitude is bound to emerge and one has to stop and 'think' about things. For example, suppose one is nursing a person diagnosed as having schizophrenia. If this person becomes agitated and disturbed, the experienced nurse simply acts. He does not reflect upon theories of the clinical care of people with schizophrenia – although he may, of course, have learned these in the past. The point is that the relevant skills can only be obtained in the relevant context, and their application does not consist in the mental rehearsal of a checklist of instructions.

CIRCUMSPECTION AGAIN

For Heidegger, circumspection is much more precise than mere manipulating and using. The nurse who is merely using and manipulating equipment needs to concentrate much more on circumspective concern. This mode of concern directs attention to relevant features of the environment:

> Rather, our concern then diverts itself specifically into a just-looking-around. But this is by no means the way in which the 'theoretical' attitude of science is reached. On the contrary, the tarrying which is discontinued when one manipulates, can take on the character of a more precise kind of circumspection, such as 'inspecting', checking up on what has been attained, or looking over the 'operations' which are now 'at a standstill'. (Heidegger, 1980, p. 409)

That is, the nurse is surveying her environment and remains bound to the practicalities of experience. Consequently, 'tarrying around' still continues when the nurse stops manipulating and using the equipment. In fact, when manipulation and using ends, circumspection becomes much more precise. We do not switch into theoretical mode and have to give a rationale for why a psychotic client is disturbed.

Rather, all the nurse does is interact with the client and use her skills and competencies, these having been derived from the past experience of similar situations. Theorising about these types of situation comes much later in the day.

Dreyfus (1991, p. 68) argues that circumspection is a mode of awareness and experience that opens up the world and the things in it, and, even though circumspection takes account of the environment without recourse to mental states, it is not mindless robotic action; it is a form of open experience rather than private subjective experience. It follows that a nurse has to take into account the surrounding practical environment of the clinical situation she is in; she has to become immersed in it to achieve a state of circumspection that is adaptable and copes with situations in a variety of ways. Dreyfus stresses that, in such coping, one responds on the basis of a vast past experience that one brings to the situation.

It is plausible to suppose that this vast array of experiences exceeds what it is possible to capture in a theory: the phenomena of coping are simply too complex. This complexity is also evident when situations in which things go wrong are considered. In such situations, the experience of the ready-to-hand environment opens up and circumspection becomes more precise.

The nurse, in order to analyse the situation by the use of circumspective penetration, plainly needs to consider the situation, but does this considering involve intentional content? Does it involve reflection upon mental representations?

It is difficult for us to pinpoint where the ontological shift from the ready-to-hand to the present-at-hand arises; that is, it is difficult to specify at what point the move from practical to theoretical thinking takes place. Heidegger does not really provide an account of this transition. However, what is important for Heidegger is that circumspection guides practice. In addition, we have to take into account that, for him:

> Circumspection operates in the involvement-relationships of the context of equipment which is ready-to-hand. Moreover, it is subordinate to the guidance of a more or less explicit survey of the equipmental totality of the current equipment-world and of the public environment which belongs to it. (Heidegger, 1980, p. 410)

Circumspection is thus subordinate to the context in which it is functioning. When the person (Dasein) surveys its whereabouts, it is locked in the totality of the equipment in which it is working. In other words, the 'equipmental totality' will determine what options are open, what it is possible for circumspection to use and manipulate. It is this environmental 'world', or context of equipment, that is the starting point for Dasein. This is what is *given* and where the human subject, Dasein, *starts* from. By analogy, this is also the starting point of the nurse in the clinical situation and should be the starting point of the curriculum.

Heidegger refines this 'surveying' of context further in this passage:

> In one's current using and manipulating, the concernful circumspection which does this 'surveying', *brings* the ready-to-hand *closer* to Dasein, and does so by interpreting what has been sighted. This specific way of bringing the object of concern close by interpreting it circumspectively, we call '*deliberating*'. (Heidegger, 1980, p. 410)

Thus 'deliberating' occurs when circumspection *interprets* an object from the relevant context and brings it to the attention of the human subject once the context (itself constituted by the 'totality of the equipment') has been 'surveyed'. Heidegger is thus opening up the ready-to-hand 'world'. This 'world' itself is claimed to be illuminated by circumspective deliberation of the environment of the ready-to-hand.

It is through circumspective deliberation that Dasein stays within the confines of the ready-to-hand and does not make an ontological shift to the theoretical present-at-hand 'world'. For Heidegger, when a breakdown of equipment occurs, circumspection 'envisages' and goes beyond the immediate context. It is a form of deliberation that takes into account what is not tangibly there. If a carpenter wants to use a nail to hang a picture on the wall, 'then' a hammer is *needed*, but if there is no hammer in the local environment, this is what happens:

> In envisaging, one's deliberation catches sight directly of that which is needed but which is un-ready-to-hand. Circumspection which envisages does not relate itself to 'mere representations'. (Heidegger, 1980, p. 410)

So even in the situation in which there is no equipment and there is a breakdown in the ready-to-hand 'world', there is, for Heidegger, still no mental representation needed to help one to make sense of the situation. What takes place is that the ready-to-hand becomes the un-ready-to-hand. When this happens, the environment announces itself as being much more complex and announces itself not as something present-at-hand nor ready-to-hand but as a social and cultural background world.

What Heidegger seems to be getting at is this. When things 'break down' or go awry, circumspection becomes more precise and takes into acount the more complex cultural background within which the inidividual is located. However, this does not yet amount to theorising. To become aware of, for example, the culture of a hospital ward, one has to be immersed in that culture. It cannot be learned from a textbook. A difficulty for us, in attempting to account for the point at which practical thinking becomes theoretical thinking, is that Heidegger seems not to provide an explanation of this process. However, one of his expositors, Dreyfus, does attempt this, and it is to his work that we now turn.

DREYFUS ON COPING AND 'BREAKDOWN'

Dreyfus attempts to describe the beginnings of the kinds of 'break-down' just referred to. He argues that it is only when things begin to break down that we switch to the subject/object mode of the present-at-hand 'world'. It is during these breakdowns that we we attempt to draw sharp divisions between ourselves and the objects that surround us. It is this switch, which Dreyfus describes, that I want to examine.

Dreyfus points out that Heidegger's new kind of intentionality, which he calls 'absorbed coping' (Dreyfus, 1991, p. 69), is not that of the Husserlian mind with a content directed towards objects. Dreyfus' problem is that Heidegger does not give an account of the emergence of the subject/object dichotomy, so he has to look for it himself. He concentrates on circumspective absorption, in which Dasein can lose itself in the world. However, it is when a breakdown occurs, such as when the head flies off the hammer or the doorknob comes off in one's hand, that traditional subject/object intentionality arises (when subjects distinguish themselves from, and reflect upon their relations to, objects):

> Once ongoing activity is held up, new modes of encountering emerge and new ways of being encountered are revealed... According to Heidegger three modes of disturbance – conspicuousness, obstinacy, and obtrusiveness – progressively bring out both Dasein as a thoughtful subject and occurrentness (present-to-hand) as the way of being of isolated, determinate substances. (Dreyfus, 1991, pp. 70–1)

In other words, all three 'modes' bring out the characteristic of the present-at-hand from what is already ready-to-hand, but what is important for Dreyfus is that when equipment malfunctions, if we can repair it or replace it very quickly, we do not begin to theorise about it. Dreyfus uses the following quote from Heidegger to support his claim:

> When its unusability is thus discovered, equipment becomes conspic-uous. This *conspicuousness* presents the ready-to-hand equipment as in

a certain un-readiness-to-hand... Pure presence-at-hand announces itself in such equipment, but only to withdraw to the readiness-to-hand of something... when we put it back into repair. (Heidegger, 1980, pp. 102–3)

Dreyfus argues that we can move into ways of coping very quickly. He gives the example of a hammer being too heavy. All we have to do is exchange it for another and we are back into the transparent coping mode very easily, all of which takes place unreflectively. It is only when the malfunction lasts and we cannot repair or replace the equipment quickly that what Dreyfus calls a *temporary breakdown* occurs; again, this is his synonym for *obstinacy*. When this happens, there is a move from absorbed coping to deliberate coping, and then to deliberation. The equipment, which was transparent when things were going smoothly, becomes explicitly manifest. It is at this point that we act *deliberately* and have to pay attention to what we are doing, says Dreyfus. We have to pay attention to the hammer and to the nails. If this *deliberate activity* of *paying attention* gets us nowhere, Dasein moves into another stance of *deliberation*, which Dreyfus argues involves reflective planning:

In deliberation one stops and considers what is going on and plans what to do, all in a context of involved activity... Deliberation can be limited to the local situation or it can take account of what is not present. Heidegger calls such long-range planning 'envisaging'. (Dreyfus, 1991, pp. 72–3)

For Dreyfus, Heidegger differs from previous philosophers in that he does not assume that mental representations are special entities in the mind that are independent of the world. As we have heard, for Heidegger, such mental items cannot be analysed without reference to the world of the thinker. Given this, Dreyfus points out that deliberation cannot be pure detached theoretical reflection for Heidegger, for such reflection always has to refer to the world, that is, to the ready-to-hand 'world'. Hence, on Dreyfus's reading of Heidegger, *deliberate action* and even theoretical contemplation take place on the background of the world. There is no mental representation or content 'in' the mind which we then act upon. Dreyfus does accept that temporary equipment breakdowns introduce mental content, but what is important is that it originates from the practical rather than the theoretical world. Consequently, circumspection can be defined as reflecting upon the experience of the practical situation of the environment of the ready-to-hand world in which the nurse dwells and is immersed; it is not a detached reflecting *away* from the ready-to-hand 'world' towards the present-at-hand theoretical 'world'.

CONCLUSION

The lesson to be learned from the above for the nurse curriculum is that attempts to elucidate the ready-to-hand world of the clinical context by the employment of present-at-hand theories are fundamentally misconceived. If Heidegger is right, such strategies get things precisely the wrong way around. For, in his account, it is the practical world, so to speak, that is the more fundamental. The skills necessary to function in that world, it appears, cannot be gleaned from the theoretical world.

For Dreyfus, the scientist dwells in the world of his discipline, which is situated in the present-at-hand world and is detached from the ready-to-hand world, but the hermeneutic ontologist dwells in the ready-to-hand world, which has a shared background understanding from which he is not detached. The latter is the nurse's position and should inform the foundation of the nurse curriculum.

REFERENCES

Benner, P. (1984) *From Novice to Expert* (Menlo Park, CA: Addison-Wesley).
Dreyfus, H.L. (1980) Holism and hermeneutics, *Review of Metaphysics*, **34**: 3–23.
Dreyfus, H.L. (1984) Introduction, in Dreyfus H.L. and Hall H. (eds) *Husserl, Intentionality, and Cognitive Science*, pp. 1–27 (Cambridge, MA: MIT Press).
Dreyfus, H.L. (1991) *Being-in-the-World: A Commentary on Heidegger's Being and Time, Division 1* (Cambridge, MA: MIT Press).
Heidegger, M. (1980, trans. J. Macquarrie and E. Robinson) *Being and Time* (Oxford: Basil Blackwell).
Heidegger, M. (1988, trans. A. Hofstadter) *The Basic Problems of Phenomenology*, (Indiana: Indiana University Press).
Magee, B. (1987) *The Great Philosophers* (London: BBC Books).
Paley, J. (1996) Intuition and expertise: comments on the Benner debate, *Journal of Advanced Nursing*, **23**: 669–72.

CHAPTER EIGHT

The unexamined life is not worth living

EDITOR'S INTRODUCTION

Janet Holt's chapter addresses a question that is fundamental to much contemporary work in nursing theory. The question concerns the status of such theories. She points out that it is common for theories of nursing to be described as 'philosophies' and moreover that such descriptions may not be wholly accurate.

According to at least one respected and plausible description of philosophy (Raphael, 1981, p. 1), it is not clear that philosophy involves the proposal of any definite claims. Rather, its concerns are more analytical. In this account, philosophy involves a process of identifying and questioning assumptions, clarifying concepts, and assessment of arguments. Furthermore, even if, within philosophy, it turns out to be the case that proposals are made, these result from the rigorous process just described.

Theories of nursing, Janet Holt suggests, fail to match the characterisation of philosophy just offered and thus only count as philosophy in an attenuated or 'non-academic' sense of that term (a 'colloquial sense', as she puts it). Basic assumptions pass unexamined (hence the chapter's title) and often unidentified. Moreover such theories are typically not subjected even to rigorous empirical enquiry.

Janet Holt's chapter prompts the following question: What is the difference, if any, between a theory of nursing, a philosophy of nursing and philosophy of nursing?

The unexamined life is not worth living

Plato, Apology, 38A

Janet Holt

Interest in the formalisation of a knowledge base in nursing has increased over the past three decades as nursing theorists have attempted to establish nursing as a practice discipline with its own knowledge base rather than one derived from social, biological and medical sciences. During this period, many theories of nursing have been developed in an attempt to explain the professional practice of nursing and differentiate between this activity and informal caring. The success of this is questionable owing to a perceived theory–practice gap. Throughout the relevant literature, there is evidence of a recurring theme that equates nursing theory with philosophy. This paper will challenge this assumption and argue that this derives from a colloquial understanding of philosophy and does not constitute a process of philosophical enquiry achieved by critical analysis of the fundamental premises on which theories rest.

PROFESSIONALISATION OF NURSING

Nursing is essentially a practical activity carried out by many people, qualified and unqualified, skilled and unskilled. A mother caring for a sick child, a practice nurse running an asthma clinic, a teenager caring for a parent with multiple sclerosis, a nurse caring for an unconscious patient with a severe head injury in ICU: in each of these cases, the person described is, broadly speaking, functioning as nurse. As the practice of nursing has moved towards professionalisation, distinctions have been made between informal and professional nursing care. Thompson et al. (1994), for example, describe three differences between professional and informal carers concerning the contractual nature of professional nursing and the relationship between the nurse and patient. A comparative analysis of informal and professional care relationships, undertaken by Kitson (1987), demonstrated similarities in commitment, sufficient levels of knowledge, skill and respect for the person by both informal and professional carers. However, professional care was sought by informal carers when they felt that their skills and knowledge were insufficient or when they became emotionally exhausted in the caring process, professional nursing care thus being a separate and more complex activity than informal caring.

A single definition of professional nursing appears to be almost enigmatic. Basford, for example, suggests that:

> professional caring is not just a reciprocal kindness, but a highly complex set of behaviours, patterns, and processes which are difficult to define. (1995, p. 107)

Irrespective of such difficulties, and of criticism of the pursuit of professionalisation from authors such as Salvage (1985), there is a desire that nursing is not simply *called* a profession but actually possesses the characteristics essential for professionalisation. Inherent in the understanding of professionalisation is the existence of a clearly defined body of knowledge. For example, a lawyer professing to be an expert in child custody would be expected to have knowledge not only of that specific area of law, but also of how to apply the law to the individual circumstances of each of her clients. Professional nursing is no exception, as embodied in the concept is the notion that professional competence is dependent upon the possession and application of knowledge unique to the discipline of nursing. There is, however, much debate over what constitutes this body of nursing knowledge. Is, for example, nursing a science or an art? What emphasis should be placed on caring? Is there indeed a unique body of knowledge, or will knowledge from other disciplines suffice? Or is nursing simply, as Draper sardonically suggests, 'those activities of health care that other workers are not interested in' (1990, p. 13).

DEVELOPMENT OF NURSING THEORY

Attempts have been made to answer such questions and others by the development of nursing theory. The drive towards professionalisation has been accompanied by the publication of several theories of nursing, mainly by North American authors. Although there are many and varied definitions of theory, theories are, broadly speaking, made up of concepts and attempt to explain the relationship and interaction between these concepts. Theories are therefore functional and tend to be constructed rather than discovered to explain phenomena. Dickoff and James describe theory as:

a conceptual system or framework invented to serve some purpose. (1968, p. 197)

They go on to describe and group different types of theory into a hierarchical framework of four levels. They suggest that nursing theory must be a theory at the highest of their four levels; such theories, they suggest, are predictive in nature. The theory for a profession such as nursing is required to do more than understand, describe and predict nursing practice but should create ideas to shape the practice of nursing. In this way, theories of nursing explain what the discipline of nursing is by organising the relationship between the concepts to describe, predict and control practice. Theories clearly need to be of benefit to the practitioner as there seems little point in developing theories of nursing that do not improve practice and enhance patient care. How successful theorists have been in their quest is open to debate, as the extensive literature on the so called theory–practice gap illustrates. Nursing theories still appear to be regarded by practitioners as episodes of academic indulgence by individuals who are unaware of the 'real world' of nursing. The sceptic may even question the need for nursing theory and view it as divorced from the practical aspects of nursing, deriding 'the academic for spinning out "mere" theories in an ivory tower' (Dickoff *et al.*, 1968, p. 418).

Practitioners may be dubious about the usefulness of theories, particularly if they lack clarity, use complex or unfamiliar language and do not appear remotely to resemble the nursing activities engaged in by practitioners. This may not necessarily be a fault of the theory but merely a problem of communicating ideas rather than the ideas themselves being flawed. However, a sceptical approach may, in itself, be useful if practitioners question the beliefs espoused by theorists and provide reasoned arguments to reject theories considered to be of limited use in practice.

PHILOSOPHY AND NURSING

Several writers equate theories of nursing with philosophies of nursing. For example, Leddy and Pepper (1993) suggest that nurses bring into practice a set of beliefs about people, the world, health and nursing that, they claim, make up a philosophy of nursing. Similarly, Cameron-Traub explains the evolution of nursing as a practice discipline in terms of philosophical perspectives on nursing practice and discipline:

Formal development of a body of nursing knowledge and theoretical expositions therein could hardly proceed without some degree of coherence in values and beliefs concerning the nature of nursing, what it is, and what it could (or should be). (1991, p. 34)

Millar (1990) describes nursing in terms of a philosophy of moral commitment whereby a nurse's personal beliefs and values about human life provide the foundation for an individual theory of nursing. Wright (1986) and Kershaw (1990) go so far as to describe nursing models as philosophies of care and suggest that a model of care is a philosophical framework for practice. Theory, philosophy and even nursing models appear to share a common meaning in the literature; this presents a confused picture to practitioners. The cause of the confusion may in part be attributed simply to this blurring of meanings, but if philosophy and theory are deemed to be synonymous, we may question whether this shared meaning also suggests a common purpose. In many other instances, this would be so. For example, I may describe a round vessel with an arched handle as a bucket or a pail; which word I choose to use may be entirely a matter of personal preference – the words are interchangeable and indicate a common purpose, that is, a vessel for carrying fluid. Similarly, if I am discussing nursing knowledge and beliefs and values about nursing, whether I choose to describe this as philosophy or theory may also be a matter of personal preference. If, however, distinctions can be drawn between the respective meanings of 'philosophy' and 'theory', they must clearly also serve different purposes.

It should be acknowledged that, unlike buckets and pails, philosophy cannot be easily defined, and, even for philosophers, its meaning is far from obvious. Philosophers such as Moore, Russell and Ayer all have difficulty in explaining exactly what philosophy is. Ayer describes the problem as follows:

What can a philosopher be said to study, in the way that a chemist studies the composition of bodies or a botanist the variety of plants? (1976, p. 1)

The preferred response of G.E. Moore to the question 'What is philosophy?' was to gesture towards his bookshelves and say, 'It is what all these are about' (Flew, 1979, p. vii).

'Philosophy' can clearly mean different things to different people at different times, but the problem concerning the provision of a definition of philosophy can be explained by drawing a distinction between two differing senses in the meaning of 'philosophy'. The first is a colloquial understanding. People often make statements beginning with the phrase 'My philosophy on life is....' This is usually followed by some description of what they 'believe in', what values they hold and what judgements they make as a result of holding these beliefs and values. For example, suppose a rock-climber is asked why she engages in a sport many would consider to be dangerous or high risk. The climber may justify her actions by saying 'My philosophy on life is "live for today".' In addition to making a positive statement about how to act, there is implicit in this statement a belief about the uncertainty of life in general and tomorrow in particular. The 'philosophy' therefore encompasses a belief regarding the uncertainty of life. This influences the actions of the climber and acts as a rationalisation for the risky behaviour. The person acknowledges the risks involved but considers such risks worth taking as there may not be another chance to do so. An understanding of 'philosophy' in this sense will be familiar to nurses engaged in writing 'unit' or 'ward' philosophies. A ward or unit philosophy usually consists of a series of statements of the beliefs held by the staff about the nature of human beings. Beliefs, for example, regarding the individual physical, psychological, social and spiritual needs of people, together with a commitment to holism, will subsequently influence the care patients can expect to receive on a particular ward or unit. Although an accepted use of philosophy, this colloquial meaning has limitations.

PHILOSOPHICAL ANALYSIS

Another understanding of philosophy is concerned less with what is said and more with what is done. Philosophy in this sense is a practical activity, one which Raphael (1981) considers to be concerned with the critical evaluation of assumptions and arguments and best understood by practical experience. Philosophy in this sense involves more than simply giving statements of one's 'beliefs' and descriptions of how such beliefs may influence behaviour. Philosophy in Raphael's sense involves examining assumptions and, more importantly, questioning the grounds for the acceptance of such assumptions. This type of philosophical analysis is crucial to nursing practice if professional nursing is to be considered as more than simply the carrying out of a series of tasks. Nursing theories and models can be used in practice in care delivery without the nurse questioning the underlying assumptions or even being convinced of their value. For example, it may be argued that a nurse may competently assess a patient, prescribe care and complete the required documentation without giving much consideration to the theory upon which the model of care is based. This is not to say that the nurse will engage in ritualistic practice and be unable to provide a rationale for care, but, in doing so, she may not necessarily question the fundamental principles upon which the model of nursing is based. Suppose a nurse is interviewed for a post on a surgical ward that uses Roy's adaptation model (Roy, 1976) to deliver nursing care. Although the nurse has no personal experience of the model, he is told by the ward manager that it is an effective way of delivering nursing care. If the nurse intends working on this ward, he will have use this model and will therefore be required to accept two assumptions: first, that Roy's model is an effective method of care delivery, and second, that physical and psychological equilibrium can be adequately explained by adaptation theory. Clearly, he can accept both assumptions without question, sign the contract and change his practice to use Roy's model. Alternatively, the assumptions can be challenged.

Raphael (1981) suggests that critical evaluation begins as a critique of assumptions, and continues by asking two further questions, namely 'Have we good reasons for accepting a belief?' and 'What are good reasons for accepting a belief?' (1981, p. 4). In the above example, the nurse will first of all need to discover good reasons for accepting the belief that Roy's model is an effective method of care delivery. To challenge this assumption, the nurse could search for evidence of empirical testing in clinical settings to support the claim. This may prove an onerous task, as Timpson (1996) suggests that nursing theories and models of nursing employed within the United Kingdom are rarely evaluated in the practice setting, either in North America or the United Kingdom. However, even if such research does exist, it will still only be of partial use in challenging the assumptions about the model. Empirical research is likely to be concerned with testing the functional role of the theory in practice rather than with the fundamental premises upon which the theory rests. This should not be interpreted as devaluing the role of empirical research in the development of nursing practice but merely as suggesting that not all questions about the nature of nursing can be answered by empirical research. The nurse may therefore find evidence to suggest that Roy's model is (or is not) an effective method of care delivery, but it is unlikely that issues regarding adaptation theory *per se* will be fully addressed.

To address these issues the nurse will need to ask Raphael's second question, 'What are good reasons for accepting a belief?', and examine the claims of adaptation theory, for example, that all human behaviour involves adaptation and that individuals react to stress through a process of adaptation. To achieve this, the nurse will probably need to read from primary sources such as Roy's original papers or even consult the writings of others such as Helson, who influenced Roy's thinking.

To challenge the assumptions in this way is to perform a critical analysis of the theory, through both the evaluation of empirical evidence and the examination of the fundamental premises upon which the theory rests, in other words to engage in philosophical enquiry.

Russell (1985) in a discussion concerning the uncertainty of philosophy, suggests that many subjects were originally part of the discipline of philosophy, but, as soon as definite knowledge about such a subject becomes evident, the subject ceases to be philosophy but instead becomes a separate science. Study of the solar system and the human mind, for example, were once the province of philosophy but have subsequently become separate disciplines. Alongside these other subjects with definite knowledge, philosophy co-exists, preoccupied with the questions that at present do not have any definite answers. For nursing, Russell's idea that subjects become separate entities is an important one. Nursing can be considered an independent discipline with – irrespective of the debate about its unique qualities – an identified body of knowledge that is nursing theory, but many other questions without definite answers still exist. For example, questions such as 'Is nursing an art or science?' or 'What is caring?' are philosophical questions rather than questions that can be completely answered by reference to nursing theory.

It may be queried whether it is necessary to go to such lengths to be a competent nurse. Can the nurse in the example above not simply agree to conform to the practices on the ward without question? The move towards professionalisation has encompassed changes in the perception of the nurses' role along with concern over the theory–practice gap. Nurses are expected to be thinking, reflective practitioners and 'knowledgeable doers', practising nurses with the ability critically to analyse knowledge and its application to modern nursing practice (UKCC, 1986). This would suggest that mere acceptance of theories of nursing without rigorous analysis is insufficient and that it would ultimately be difficult to distinguish between this form of nursing practice and the largely discredited ritualised care practised in earlier decades. This can in part be addressed by the examination of empirical evidence, but critical analysis of the fundamental premises of nursing theory is as necessary as evaluation of the functional elements of the theory.

To describe nursing theory as a philosophy of nursing is to demonstrate nothing more than a colloquial understanding of the term 'philosophy'. Philosophy can be understood as being quite separate from nursing theory, nursing models or even a ward or unit philosophy by drawing a clear distinction between the purpose of philosophical enquiry and the purpose of nursing theory. It is clearly necessary to identify a starting point, which is usually the position taken by theorists who make statements about the beliefs and values they hold. These may be expressed through some form of conceptual framework, such as the nursing metaparadigm, and theories may be advanced relating to beliefs held about the concepts of person, environment, health and nursing. The function of the theory is to inform, provide a rationale for and enhance practice, and ultimately improve patient care, in short, to be of use to nurses and to benefit patients. To develop nursing theory for reasons other than these would be a worthless activity. However, instead of accepting theories as self-evident truths, nurses need critically to evaluate theory and consider whether they have good reasons to pay heed to the ideas. If the nurse finds that there do not appear to be good reasons for accepting the claims, the theory should then be rejected and alternatives sought. Thus, for example, if a theory advances a claim concerning individuals or nursing practice, the theory should be examined by questioning whether it is true, why it should be believed, why it should be trusted over other, possibly contradictory, theories and what evidence there is to support the proposals made in the theory. If theories of nursing are considered to be synonymous with philosophies of nursing, critical evaluation of the beliefs and arguments that underpin the theory is, by definition, necessary as part of the development process.

During the past 30 years, progress has been made in explaining the discipline of nursing through the use of nursing theories. Definitions of theory encompass functional elements by suggesting that theories exist for some purpose which, in nursing, relates to caring for patients. The integration of theory and practice is not without difficulty, and practitioners may be reluctant to accept such ideas as being relevant to their practice. This reluctance tends to have a negative focus, which in many instances may be justified. However, scepticism is itself not necessarily detrimental to nursing practice. Throughout the literature, nursing theory is considered to be synonymous with philosophy. As noted, this involves a colloquial understanding of philosophy rather than a process of philosophical inquiry derived from critical analysis of the fundamental premises on which the theory rests: 'Philosophy is not a theory but an activity [which aims at the] logical clarification of thoughts' (Wittgenstein, 1922, para. 4.112).

REFERENCES

Ayer, A.J. (1976) *The Central Questions of Philosophy* (Harmondsworth: Penguin).

Basford, L. (1995) Professional care, in Basford, L. and Slevin, O., *Theory and Practice of Nursing*, pp. 106–14 (Edinburgh: Campion Press)

Cameron-Traub, E. (1991) An evolving discipline, in Gray, G. and Pratt, R. (eds) *Towards a Discipline of Nursing*, (Melbourne: Churchill Livingstone) pp. 31–49.

Dickoff, J. and James, P. (1968) A theory of theories: a position paper, *Nursing Research*, **17**(3): 197–203.

Dickoff, J., James, P. and Weidenbach E. (1968) Theory in a practice discipline. Part 1. Practice orientated theory, *Nursing Research*, **17**(5): 415–35.

Draper, P. (1990) The development of theory in British nursing: a current position and future prospects, *Journal of Advanced Nursing*, **15**: 12–15.

Flew, A. (1979) *A Dictionary of Philosophy* (London: Pan).

Helson, H. (1964) *Adaptation-Level Theory: An Experimental and Systematic Approach To Behaviour* (New York: Harper & Row).

Kershaw, B. (1990) Nursing models as philosophies of care, *Nursing Practice*, **4**(1): 25–7.

Kitson, A. (1987) Raising standards of clinical practice; the fundamental issue of effective nursing practice, *Journal of Advanced Nursing*, **12**: 321–9.

Leddy, S. and Pepper, J.M. (1993) *Conceptual Bases of Professional Nursing*, 3rd edn (Philadelphia: JB Lippincott).

Millar, B. (1990) The benefits of nursing models, *Surgical Nurse*, **3**(1): 5–8.

Raphael, D.D. (1981) *Moral Philosophy* (Oxford: Oxford University Press).

Roy, C. (1976) *Introduction to Nursing: An Adaptation Model* (Englewood Cliffs, NJ: Prentice-Hall).

Salvage, J. (1985) *The Politics of Nursing* (London: Heinemann).

Russell, B. (1985) *The Problems of Philosophy* (Oxford: Opus).

Thompson, I.E., Melia, K. and Boyd, K.M. (1994) *Nursing Ethics*, 3rd edn (Edinburgh: Churchill Livingstone).

Timpson, J. (1996) Nursing theory: everything the artist spits is art?, *Journal of Advanced Nursing*, **23**: 1030–6.

UKCC (1986) Project 2000: *A New Preparation to Practice* (London: UKCC).

Wittgenstein, L. (1922) *Tractatus-Logico-Philosophicus* (London: Routledge & Kegan Paul).

Wright, S. (1986) *Building and Using a Model of Nursing* (London: Edward Arnold).

Part IV

THE SELF IN NURSING

The self

Paul Dawson's ambitious chapter describes the transition from the adoption of a Cartesian view of the self to that of a narrative view of the self. The Cartesian view is said to have been characteristic of the 'modern' era while the narrative view is characteristic of the 'post-modern' era.

The importance of the conception of the self to nursing is particularly pertinent, although not exclusively so, to mental health nursing – Dawson's particular field of expertise. For example, suppose it is true, as he suggests, that selves are 'socially constructed'. It seems to follow from this that, in psychiatric care, it will be essential to take into account the client's cultural background. This may not even be possible for carers who have a cultural heritage different from that of the client. Clearly, this point can be generalised to apply to all types of nursing and to midwifery. Moreover, Dawson suggests that the theory and practice of psychiatry presuppose a Cartesian conception of the self; this is typically appealed to in the concept of the 'ego'. Such a Cartesian view of the self, Dawson argues, is open to serious objection. If he is right about both of these claims, therapeutic regimes based on the Cartesian view will be theoretically unfounded. For example, suppose he is right that the purported aim of much psychiatric care is to 'salvage the self' or ego, and that the self is typically construed as a Cartesian self. How might one go about salvaging the 'unitary' self or ego – given that there is no such thing?

The view of the self that Dawson favours is a narrative view. In brief, this holds that there is no continuous 'unitary' self. Instead, there are held to be a succession of selves constituted by overlapping narratives. In this conception, the subject of mental experience – the thinker – seems to evaporate.

It should be stressed that consideration of the concept of the self is not of relevance solely to those interested in mental health issues (as Dawson makes clear). The chapter explains that if selves are to be construed as 'narratives', the concept of the self will contain an inescapable cultural element. As noted above, it follows from this that nursing people from cultures other than one's own may well prove to be problematic. For example, the possibility arises of a culture in which the idea of an 'autonomous self' does not have the central role it is accorded in Western cultures. Where this is the case, it could be expected that much less importance will be attached to 'respecting the autonomy' of patients and clients. Hence, Dawson's chapter points to an important problem for any approach to nursing practice and nursing ethics that emphasises the importance of respecting autonomy.

Regardless of the last point, it is clear that there are many situations within general nursing, children's nursing and midwifery in which the concept of self is problematic. Such situations include the peri- and post-operative contexts, and also perinatal contexts. Can patients and clients in these contexts give voice to 'what they really want' or is the integrity of the self overwhelmed in such contexts – perhaps by stress, anxiety and the effects of medication? Also, of course, conditions such as multiple sclerosis, kidney disease and heart disease are each plausibly regarded as having such a deep impact upon their sufferers that the very nature of the self is challenged. Dawson's chapter has ramifications for all these issues.

The self

Paul Dawson

others made me, and continue to make me the person I am (Sandel, 1982, p. 143)

One of the prime psychological ingredients of an individual's interpretation of the behavioural environment, particularly in Western cultures, is the concept of an autonomous self. The self can be defined in general terms as an individual that is conscious of the individual that it is while at the same time being conscious that it is the individual it is conscious of (Priest, 1991). The concept of the self is, therefore, inextricably interwoven with concepts of mind and of consciousness.

It is fair to say that the self and its attributes have been most closely studied by the disciplines of psychology and philosophy. In modern psychology, the prevailing tendency has been to treat the self as an unchangeable, transhistorical entity (a unified core self), a datum of existence which it is the goal of psychology to describe in all its manifestations. Philosophical approaches to the question of the self, on the other hand, tend to put in question the very data that support the psychological viewpoint. Philosophers are primarily concerned with the self as it is revealed by conscious introspection.

In recent times, psychology has developed a renewed interest in the ontological foundations of the self. This has re-awakened the historical alliance between philosophy and psychology, which dates back to the early Greek philosophers. The impetus behind this revival may be traced to the reconceptualisations of the concept of self necessitated by two kinds of enquiry in philosophy, each of which questions the whole idea of unity and foundations. The first line of enquiry is that conducted by Jacques Derrida and the philosophy of post-modernism.[1] The second line of enquiry derives from recent attempts to model the mind in computer terms (connectionism).[2] Each of these two approaches has tended to highlight the problems surrounding our concepts of language, memory and perception.

These are plausibly seen as the basis of our capacity for reflective thought, and without which, it seems, there would be no concept of self in the first instance.

In what follows, I will attempt to describe the nature of the threat posed by these developments in thought about the self to a Cartesian conception of the self, which is widely prevalent in nursing and in Western thought generally. The early sections of the chapter set out the Cartesian view, report its influence and consider criticisms posed for it. Later sections attempt to elaborate a conception of the self that is radically different from the Cartesian view; the new, radical conception can be said to adopt a 'narrative' conception of the self. However, for now, I begin with some brief remarks that attempt to make clear the relevance of this discussion to nursing. In a later section, I discuss in greater depth the implications that conceptions of the self carry for psychiatric nursing.

THE SELF IN NURSING

Why is the self such an important concept in nursing? When we consider the nature of mental disorder, the most striking and consistent feature reported is a changed concept of the self. A frequent complaint from families and relatives trying to make sense of the changes occurring to their son or daughter, for example, is that they are no longer their usual self, that they have, in effect, become a stranger. This is the objective perception or view from the third-person perspective. Subjectively, from the first-person perspective, the person suffering from a mental disorder experiences a disruption in his or her sense of self. In psychosis, for example, the notion of a controlling self, an 'I' who thinks thoughts and is the doer of actions, is often lost. Thoughts become alien, no longer authored by the putative subject. Instead, the thoughts are experienced as 'not mine' but as somehow put there by another. In terms we shall consider shortly, the subject is no longer the author of the ongoing narrative of his or her self. In depressive states, one can come to despise the self that one presently 'has', or in states of mania, aggrandise oneself beyond reason.

In physical disorders, too, the subject may experience a disruption of the sense of self. The experience of major surgery or of treated cardiac arrest, for example, can often lead to a major re-evaluation of the sense of self and self-worth as one learns to live with loss and impairment. How is one changed, for example, by loss of a limb or an organ, and by the realisation that the body is no longer subject to the will? These brief considerations indicate the importance and centrality of the concept of the self as it applies to the context of nursing theory and practice.

THE CARTESIAN SELF

Generally speaking, the conception of the self most commonly encountered in nursing theory, and in psychology and psychiatry, is essentially Cartesian in nature. The philosophy of Rene Descartes (1596–1650) represents a watershed in Western thinking on the nature of the self. Descartes liberated the rational aspect of humankind from the confines of the body, thus clearing the way for the reconceptualisation of the body in purely physical and mechanical terms. In his 'Sixth Meditation', Descartes insists on his nature as 'a conscious, not an extended [material] being'. The body, in contrast, is conceived of as 'extended' and without consciousness (1970, p. 114). Descartes concluded, 'I am really distinct from my body, and could exist without it' (1970, p. 115).

Descartes derived his claims from what was revealed to him by introspection. He discovered that, although he could doubt most things, he could not doubt that he was doubting and that he was conscious of doubting. This led to Descartes' famous dictum 'I think, therefore I am' (1970, p.183). Moreover, Descartes' deliberations set in motion a dualist conception of the nature of human beings, the influence of which on Western thought has been far reaching and profound.

Having thus separated mind and body, Descartes proposed a meeting point in the pineal gland of the brain, a central point where mind and body come together, a seat of consciousness. It is here that the 'ego' or self, as conceived of by Descartes, exerts control over the body. Thus, in Cartesian terms, when we say 'I', we are referring to a particular *thing*, to a self or ego inhabiting the body but essentially different from that body.

However, the properties that Descartes ascribed to the self are, on further examination, not quite so evident. If we ask ourselves exactly what 'I' refers to, we seem to find that it refers to nothing apart from a stream of mental experiences. That is to say, when we introspect, we do not seem to encounter a thing called the self. We encounter only our thoughts and experiences, the thoughts and experiences of a self. Furthermore, exactly what 'I' is taken to refer to is dependent in a general sense on the context (it depends on who is presently speaking), and in a more particular sense on whether a self is to be thought of as a person's body or brain, or as a Cartesian soul or ego.

In Western psychological theory, the legacy of Descartes has been to reify consciousness as an ego, separated from the material world. As such, it is only contingently related to the world. This view of the self as a *thing*, the *object* of introspection, has given rise to the effort to frame psychological science in terms of the natural sciences. Human action is reduced to the necessarily lawful outcomes of the physical *processes* inherent in the person. This has resulted in a tendency to disregard the social role of the person and the environment in the genesis and treatment of psychological maladies.

This 'decontextualisation' of the self trades upon a particular conception of causal relations. It is one according to which 'internal' events determine behaviour. This way of construing the causes of behaviour has been partly responsible for the increasing emphasis in current psychiatric research on the biological basis of mental disorder.

THE FREUDIAN SELF

When we consider theories of the self in the context of nursing, they are invariably based on the notions of ego psychology, and carry into the body of nursing theory all the intellectual baggage of Cartesianism. Freudian theory, whose influence in one guise or another is pervasive in most nursing texts, may be said to straddle the divide between the neurologically founded experience of the person and the structures of the human world.

There is, in Freud's work, a persistent tension between an inherently Cartesian first-person theory of consciousness and a nascent interpersonal view of the self. (By an 'interpersonal' view of the self, I mean a view of the self in which the very concept of the self requires reference to other selves.) The Cartesian commitment is evident in the following quote: 'our assumption of a consciousness [in other men] rests upon an inference and cannot share the immediate certainty which we have of our own consciousness' (Freud, 1963, p. 169). Evidence of a nascent interpersonal model can be gleaned from the claim, inherent in the Oedipal theory, that identification with others is necessary in forming a system of values. One can note also the emphasis in Freud's practice on interpretation and dialogue, the sharing of a common language and the importance of transference and countertransference *relationships*.

Later developments in the view of the self prevalent in psychoanalytic theory broadened the notion of self, moving from the self seen simply as the sum of the content of the mental apparatus, or the outcome of drive cathexes, to a view of the self as the *centre* of the psychological universe. Therapy then becomes the process of analysis and development of the self so constructed.

The thrust in modern psychoanalytic interpretation has been to move towards an analysis of the self in terms of the whole person's subjective experience and the person's sense of self as derived from the relations with others. This is in contradiction to Freud's classical model. However, both positions (ego/self analyses) nevertheless retain the presumption of an 'entity' within the mind that functions as the guarantor of psychic wholeness, this entity being the self or the ego.

The self takes many guises in psychoanalytic theory, from that which is dependent on identification with others – Freud's superego – through to Kohut's (1977) 'nuclear' self and Kernberg's (1982) analysis of the self in terms of an enduring kernel of ego structures underlying constant patterns of behaviour. All of these revisions of Freudian theory that posit some variety of the unified self are, in varying degrees, contrary to Freud's own position in which the multiplication of structural phenomena within the mind paints a picture of a mind and a self constitutionally divided. The aim of Freud's therapy is to re-integrate the parts of the self cut or split off from the conscious self, to restore wholeness, in Freud's famous dictum, to ensure that 'Where Id was, there Ego shall be' or 'Where It was, there I shall be' (1933, p. 80).

THE LACANIAN SELF

One of the more radical revisions of Freud, whose influence is not yet evident in nursing texts, is that of Jacques Lacan (1901–81). In this, the Freudian ego is recast as a *misrecognition* of what is. Freud's theory was based on the conception of the ego as a controller who modulates the excesses of the Id's unthinking pursuit of immediate pleasure – rather as a horseman might strive to control a frisky stallion. The ego here *is* the conscious self, the pilot at the helm. In the Lacanian formulation, the ego is an *imaginary* synthesis, formed between the ages of 6 and 18 months in response to the reflected image of the infant in a mirror. The stable selfhood of this reflected image is in marked contrast to the infant's undeveloped motor capacity and its helpless dependence on others.

Before acquiring language, and in the absence of any other social determinant, the self is constituted as both a fiction (the unattainable wholeness of the mirror image) and a source of alienation (the self as other, an objective image). In the mirror image, the infant misrecognises himself, says Lacan, and in this misrecognition lies the source of all future aggressivity, as the unified and whole mirror image is constituted as a superior and rival self to the as yet undifferentiated infant. Thus, Lacan concludes, aggressivity, rivalry, ambivalence and identification with others are all *preceded* by the structure of the self relationship.

Lacan posits the self as resulting from an originary split (the misidentification of the self as the mirror image); this has the consequence that the subject is 'born divided'. The illusory unity of the reflected image is always luring the subject away from him or herself. Lacan's ideas in this respect, principally the misidentification of the self with an imaginary construct, share many affinities with the thought of Jean-Paul Sartre (1905–80).

THE SARTREAN SELF

Sartre was of the opinion that Western thought had been led astray by the idea that the reflecting consciousness (the thinker) and the reflected consciousness (the object of thought) are in some way different. In Descartes, as we have seen, this results in the conception of an immaterial but substantial unitary self, separate from the body and transparent to processes of rational enquiry. However, in Sartre's view, the positing of both a reflecting and a reflected consciousness, upon which the reflecting consciousness focuses as a mental object or idea, gives rise to the concept of a reified ego or self separate from the world, which is *taken to be consciousness*.

In this process, the reflecting consciousness disappears from view. The reflected consciousness is mistaken for consciousness *per se* (the reified ego), the reflecting consciousness itself in turn standing in need of reflection. Pursuing this course involves an infinite regress as each (mental) object for a subject (reflected consciousness for a reflecting consciousness) leaves the subject as unknown and as unknowable as before, hence Sartre's characterisation of the concept of the ego as 'a perpetually deceptive mirage' (1957, p. 69).

THE SELF RECONSIDERED

The notion, then, that it is psychologically advantageous to have a strong ego, a foundation stone of Freudian thought, is cast into serious doubt by both these thinkers. For them, the ego is a fictive, imaginary construct of consciousness, constituting a misrepresentation or misrecognition of what is. To reinforce the power of this deceptive mirage over an already riven and alienated subject is only to compound the problem.

While there are points of agreement in Sartre and Lacan, Lacan strongly criticises Sartre's continuing insistence on the privileging of the subject. For Lacan, Sartre remains within the limits of a self-sufficiency of consciousness, which effectively dismisses the role of the other (that is, other people or selves) in the constitution of the subject. While the mirror stage, like Sartre's reflecting/reflected polarity, is still fundamentally solipsistic, Lacan further developed the notion of the self in terms of the self's introduction to speech and language and encounters with other selves, a point we return to later. Such ideas (ideas that undermine the legitimacy of a 'pure' Cartesian self) lead to several interrelated conclusions concerning the self and the possibility of self-knowledge. The self constituted in this fashion cannot give us access to self-knowledge for a number of reasons.

First, as we have seen, the self is a *construct* of consciousness and is not to be confused with either consciousness itself or the subject. Second, our experience of the self as somehow 'inside' us is an illusion caused by our innate tendency to reverse the real order of things. This results in our attributing behaviour to a substantive self or ego rather than seeing the *concept* of self and ego as a product of such behaviour. If, as Sartre has sought to demonstrate, the self is an object in the external world (a reified, reflected ego), and for Lacan a misrecognition founded on the illusion of unity, the insights of introspection are of necessity false. Finally, introspection *per se*, in the absence of a relatedness to an external world, necessarily leads to the paradoxes of solipsism and the complete loss of the self. Indeed, it can be argued that the loss of the self characteristic of schizophrenic illness, for example, is a product of *excessive* introspection, of a hyper-rationality, which in its continual objectification of subjective experience serves to undermine the sense of self. The often observed clinical fact that such symptoms as auditory hallucinations are exacerbated in intensity by social isolation and inactivity (in which the opportunities for 'morbid' introspection are intensified), yet diminish in parallel with increasing activity and socialisation, lend some support to this view.

THE POST-INDIVIDUALISTIC, NARRATIVE SELF

The dominant Western psychological models of the self maintain the notion of an internal locus of control, with well-defined boundaries between the self and the not-self. This conception survives in spite of the 'decentreing' of the self inherent in Freud's model and the revisionist promptings of Lacan and Sartre (Baumeister, 1987). As one of the pre-established categories around which we construct our view of the world, the hypothesis of a unitary self has now become part of our cultural and intellectual inheritance. Developed during the era of modernism, it was formulated in terms of the framework of understanding particular to that era (Sampson, 1988). The present era is post-industrial and information-based, and it may well be that the concept of self that is characteristic of the modern age of industrialisation and individualism has outlived its utility. The concept of the self that is currently being elaborated in our era, the *post-modern* era, emphasises the decentred nature of the self, the absence of a unitary Cartesian controller or ego. In the new conception, relatedness takes precedence over unity and mastery. Self-identity, in the new paradigm, 'is constituted and reconstituted relationally, its boundaries repeatedly recomposed and renegotiated' (Scott, 1987, p. 17).

In part, this re-conceptualising of the self springs from the changing scientific perception of the world. The static Newtonian world-view that gave rise to the Western concept of the self has ceded to a more dynamically oriented conception, a world of process in continual flux. Indeed, the world of modern physics seems more akin to the world of Buddhist philosophy, in which things and substance are viewed as 'samsara', that is, as 'deeds or events' (Suzuki, 1968, p. 55). Reality is now sought in relation rather than in substance. Selfhood thus does not derive its order from its presumed attributes of unity and integration, but rather from being '[A] continuously evolving process, whose evolvingness rather than its thinghood is its very essence' (Sampson, 1985, p. 1206).

In this post-modern re-ordering of the intellectual world, narrative assumes great importance (see Sarbin, 1986). Story-telling (narrative) and propositional thinking (argumentation) provide distinctive alternative means for the ordering of experience. Narrative is concerned with the particular, the contextual, and with the intentions and actions of humans. Propositional thinking, on the other hand, seeks to transcend the particular or contextual in search of increasing levels of abstraction.

From the perspective of post-modern thought, the inner world of experience is a kind of 'telling' rather than a place. Hermans *et al.* (1992, p. 28) have conceptualised this narrative self as dialogical, that is, 'in terms of a dynamic multiplicity of relatively autonomous I positions in an imaginal landscape'. The 'I' endows each position with a voice, enabling dialogical relations to be established between them, each position functioning as a character in the story of the self. The differing stories that the 'I' positions relate about 'me' (the actor in the real world) constitute the complex of the narratively structured self. In contrast to the individualistic self of Cartesianism, the 'I' occupies many positions from which it can agree or disagree with other 'I' positions. Any 'I' position may at any time become an anchor point around which the others may become temporarily organised in a continual interchange.

The notion of a dominant 'I' position, an ego, an individualised self, is presumed to arise through cultural and educational constraints, which serve to force the polyphonic chorus of the self into a muted individualistic performance. Among such constraints, we may include the pervasive influence of Freudian ego psychology in a society that is dedicated to economic productivity and the promotion of mass consumerism as the royal road to happiness.

The dialogical self (or selves) is dependent on language rather than mental mechanisms for its expression, the same language, which, for Lacan, is a vehicle of cultural conditioning and the precondition for awareness of oneself as a separate being.[3] The general movement of thought is from private to public meaning, from the private cabinet of Cartesian consciousness locked in one's head, to consciousness and self constituted in the public arena of language.

Lacan's objection to ego psychology has two dimensions. First is the tendency to downplay the role of language and to emphasise developmental psychology at the expense of this linguistic dimension (an emphasis particularly prevalent in nursing texts). Second is the predilection for quasi-scientific alienating objectifications, which reproduce in the therapeutic setting precisely that objectification of the subject which it is the purpose (?) of therapy to counteract. This has the effect of re-stating conformity to the prevailing cultural *status quo* as mental health (in nursing texts, this point of view is almost universal). Lacan puts it thus:

> For if [the ego's] health is defined by its adaptation to a reality that is regarded *quite simply as being suited to it*, and if you need the cooperation of the 'healthy part of the ego' in order to reduce, in the other part no doubt, incompatibilities with reality... is it not clear that there is no

other way of distinguishing the healthy part of the subject's ego than by its *agreement with your point of view*... just as there is *no other criterion of cure than the complete adoption by the subject of this measure of yours*... (1977, p. 135, emphases added)

Psychiatric nursing, we may note, is sometimes *defined* as the therapeutic use of self (see Stuart and Sundeen, 1991, p. 26), in which the nurse has an 'obligation to model adaptive and growth producing behaviour', such behaviour being implicitly defined as that which accords with cultural norms.

The assumption that mental health is to be equated with compliance to social norms, in the absence of any critique or justification of these norms, lays the groundwork for the abuse of psychiatric powers for which the former Soviet Union was so roundly criticised. In Western society, the fear of the instinct-driven, potentially dangerous self, has been used by the state to justify its role in the control and regulation of the self. However, the role of mental health professionals in the exercise of this control has been equally enthusiastic. (I remember with chagrin the accusation hurled at me by a patient in an English psychiatric hospital some years ago: 'You're just another of the psychiatric thought police!')

THE CONNECTIONIST SELF[2]

Some interesting points of correspondence have recently begun to emerge between modern computer modelling of the brain's activities and post-modern views of the nature of the self. The tendency to ask what the self is poses the question in a metaphysical form, inviting the response that the self is a substance (a thing), which somehow supports or is the source of all the activities that selves are supposed to engage in. One would expect this mysterious thing to have some neural counterpart, some grouping of executive neurones within the brain that could be identified as the seat of action of the self. (Freud, in his *Project for a Scientific Psychology*, 1895, for example, went so far as to sketch the neural make-up of the ego.) This 'soul pearl', as Dennett calls it (1991, p. 423), this highly specialised group of neurones, would *be* the self and would control all 'selfy' activities.

With commendable prescience, given the direction of future enquiries, James (1890, p. 180) also pointed out that no group of cells within the brain could be considered the keystone or centre of gravity of the whole system. The notion of control in this sense is entirely lacking from modern connectionist modelling of neural events, in which activation states settle out from the general neural activity in accordance with the degree of disorder of the system, the process favouring states of low statistical energy. The whole system (the mind/brain) proceeds, then, by a process in accord with *statistical laws*, and there is no specific brain area that can be considered the final arbiter of such information processing. Rather than a centre of control (the conscious self) coordinating the expression of these various states, all states are in competition for expression.[4] Whichever state succeeds is a product of several factors operative in the system as a whole, including some 'hard wired' weightings (for example, pain will receive preferential attention) and the degree of concordance with some other weighted models of the world and the self.

THE MEADIAN SELF

Rather than specify the self in this fashion, that is, in terms of process (the 'what' of the self), post-modern thought concentrates on the 'how' of the self – self as activity. A much-negelected precursor of this approach is the social psychologist George Herbert Mead (1863–1931). Mead considered the self to be a *product* of social behaviour rather than some mysterious entity inhabiting the psyche and *producing* such behaviour; he asserted that the self (and, indeed, mind) evolves in processes of social interaction. Essential to such processes are the institutions of organised society, which reflect the general social life process and without which, in Mead's view, there could be no fully mature individual selves at all. The post-modern re-evaluation of the self likewise re-inserts the abstract notion of the self into its cultural and social context.

In contrast, modernist theory, upon which much psychiatric and psychological research is based, attempts to abstract a notional 'self' from its context. The real, the 'true', self is to be found by stripping away the social roles and revealing the inner, private experiences that constitute this self. These experiences themselves may then be recast in terms of neural functions. However, as James (1890) pointed out, the person (as opposed to such reductionist subsystems) appears as both partly known and partly knower, partly object and partly subject, the 'I' experiencing both the outer world and the 'me', the objectively known sum of a person's knowledge and awareness. The 'I', in James's view, is a process, the ongoing stream of (self) consciousness.

The influence of Freudian thought, and the modern ego psychology to which it gave birth, has served to downplay the cultural and social context and to emphasise the necessity of strengthening the ego (conceived of as an intrapsychic mechanism or homunculus) in achieving wellness. This is also the consistent stance of many of the techniques standardly advocated in psychiatric nursing textbooks, with their emphasis on the therapeutic use of the self. The assumption is that this self is bounded, unitary and masterful in the classical Cartesian sense. Yet if the autonomous, bounded self or ego is an illusion, a socially, culturally and historically conditioned construct, what are we to make of these therapies, based as they are on a possibly outmoded and static construct of the self? Are they likewise dangerous and misleading?

THE SELF IN PSYCHIATRIC NURSING

Lather (1992) comments on the manner in which language can create areas of silence by organising meaning in terms of pre-established categories. These lacunae, these absences in a discourse, serve to protect the *status quo* from unsettling critical analysis. In the discourse of psychiatric nursing texts, there is a large lacuna of silence surrounding the notion of self. This absence is sometimes obscured by the voluminous entries in the indexes of such texts under self-concept, self-esteem, self-care, self-destruction and so on. On close examination, however, it becomes evident that, typically, there are no entries under the concept of the self itself. Presumably this is because the nature of the self is deemed transparent to the authors of such texts and to the expected audience. A random sampling of currently used texts reveals that the concept of self presumed is that which we have typified as unitary, individualistic and masterful. It is a basically Freudian or ego psychological model developing through distinct stages to a position of maturity and 'inside' the person in some sense: the prevalent Western cultural stereotype.

Arthur *et al.* (1992), for example, utilise Freud, Rogers and Maslow, and in particular the notion of self-actualisation, which implies that there is a true self that needs to be actualised: 'by the implementation and realisation of a person's true potential' (Stuart and Sundeen, 1991, p. 376). Most texts agree that realisation of this potential is dependent on the existence of 'certain elements of ego strength [which] provide a foundation on which to build' (Stuart and Sundeen, 1991, p. 399). The concept of the ego (or self) is itself never subjected to any critique or interrogation.

The basic premise of many of the therapeutic techniques advocated is that the disturbances in the self of the mentally ill person represent a falling away from the idealised norm. Such disturbances are claimed to be manifested in a loss of control, in a loss of agency and in aberrant perceptions of the self. The closer these aberrant perceptions are to 'the core of the self concept, the more difficult [they are] to change' (Stuart and Sundeen, 1995, p. 398). Change, in this context, means reinforcing the culturally acceptable self. A person with a weak or negative self concept, for example is described as 'likely to have narrowed or distorted perceptions', while a person with a strong or positive self concept 'can explore his world openly and honestly because he has a background of acceptance and success' (Stuart and Sundeen, 1991, p. 377). The normative and evaluative elements in such statements are revealing.

From a differing perspective (say, that of Lacan), as we have seen, appeals to such a concept of the self may amount to building illusory castles in the air. In terms of the narrative conception of the self, such a strategy merely serves to *arrest* the development of complementary or antagonistic 'I' positions by strengthening one (the ego as master) at the expense of many others. Again, the unity is illusory. The achievement of the person's 'true potential' is invariably couched in terms of achieving autonomy, control, individualisation and integration, thus normalising behaviour in terms of culturally accepted standards. I have failed to find any appreciation in the nursing texts of the sources and nature of these standards, nor any appreciation of their cultural relativity.

While the thrust of more recent reconceptualisations of the self has been to unshackle the concept from its Cartesian roots, the view promulgated in nursing texts, with the emphasis on the tenets of ego psychology, is curiously reactionary. The mental world portrayed is suffocating in its neatness and order, constrained, regimented and regulated. It is as though a whole area of critical discourse has passed unnoticed, as though James had never delivered his scathing verdict on the concept of the ego as 'only a cheap and nasty edition of the soul... simply *nothing*; as ineffectual and windy an abortion as philosophy can show' (1890, vol. 1, p. 365). What, then, is one to make of the demand to use the 'ego strengths' of the individual in therapy, the same ego which Lacan criticised as being *the root cause of mental disturbance*, and as 'the centre of all resistances' (1977, p. 23)?

CONCLUSION

The wisdom of the emphasis placed in nursing texts on ego psychology is open to serious question. There is a clear need for more discussion of alternative theoretical positions, especially given the many doubts that surround the Cartesian bias implicit in appeals to the ego. The concept of individuality we currently have, the form of subjectivity sanctioned by culture and society may no longer be adequate. Also, as Foucault (1980, p. 216) suggests, the time may be ripe for the refusal of present forms of subjectivity and the promotion of new forms. The emphasis in nursing texts on reinforcing ego strengths may be seen as promoting the view that therapy means adjustment rather than change, of insisting on the primacy of the concept of the autonomous self and of shying away from the necessarily revolutionary implications of alternative conceptualisations.

In the traditional sense, as a central controlling agent, the ego or self *does not exist*. It is not a substance or thing (soul/ego) that in some way *pre-exists* speech or thought as the place from which one speaks. Rather, it is produced by the social interactions among persons as mediated by both language and the institutions of society. As such, it does not reside inside the person in some mysterious fashion. The post-modern view of the self eschews individualism and rationality (the bulwarks of modern industrial society) in favour of an embodied social self that incorporates the other in the self. Hence, the idea arises of there being a multiplicity of 'selves', a multiplicity of 'I' positions. Such a self is conceived of as a self that is perennially in progress, with no fixed identity. The operational logic of the post-modern self runs contrary to the either/or binarism of rational thought. The axiomatic assumptions underlying theory in most nursing texts are structured by such binarism, the dysjunction between, in crude terms, the sane and insane, the healthy and the unhealthy, identity and fragmentation, self and not-self. From either side of these polarities, the position of the other is incomprehensible. To the mad, we appear equally mad.

Each of us is an agent with an identity, but the tendency we have noted in Western thought to posit a further agent within (an ego, a 'soul pearl') is unnecessary. The thoughts that represent models of the self to the thinker, the 'me' of Mead and James, are in a sense things seen rather than the seer. The seer itself may be thought of as the whole organism complete with functional nervous system, as Flanagan (1994) suggests.

When we use the indexical term 'I', we may be referring to the organism that is doing the thinking or to some model of the self, or to one of the 'mes' that is constituted by the internalised attitudes of others – for example, in the processes of socialisation and interaction. When 'I' is used in this latter narrow sense, it refers to a particular self in a particular context – my 'professional' self, my 'musical' self, my 'psychotic' self – each of which may be viewed as an aspect of an ongoing narrative construction that is subject to radical change over time. The elements of this narrative are essentially individual in their particulars, although the framework in which they are placed is a product of social conditioning. There is thus an inherent ambiguity in the self, in that the very social structures which give the individual a shape and the possibility of expression, at one and the same time constrain and limit both feelings and expression. Changes in these social structures will, in this view, necessarily be reflected in changes in the concept of the self. In a society increasingly oriented towards production and consumerism, which valorises a spurious individuality over the values of community and sociality, and in which the person is reduced to a 'dehumanised functionary' (Zidjerveld, 1974, p. 80), it should come as no surprise that the concept of self is undergoing radical revision. How these revisions are effected, which comes to hold sway in our model of self, will have far reaching implications, both for society at large and for psychiatric nursing in particular.

NOTES

1. Post-modernism, in the sense used in this chapter, refers to a branch of thought reflecting present-day disbelief in the meta-narratives (scientific and philosophical) that formerly structured our (modern) view of the world. With this disbelief comes an emphasis on heterogeneous and local narratives, as opposed to homogeneous and universal narratives, and a move from the search for eternal and immutable truths to an acceptance of the chaotic, ephemeral, discontinuous and fragmented nature of reality.
2. Connectionism (also known as parallel distributed processing – PDP) refers to a particular computer modelling of the brain processes involved in cognition. Typically, a connectionist system is composed of a number of units, which, like neurones, are activated to a greater or lesser degree. The degree of activation of any unit can act to increase or decrease the activation of those other units to which it is connected, such activation being subject to variation over time. When the system is activated (presented with a 'problem'), it eventually settles into a stable state such that further activation does not lead to subsequent change in the activation strength of the component units. This settled state is the 'solution' to the presenting problem. See P. Churchland and T.J. Sejnowski, Neural representation and neural computation, and W. Bechtel, Connectionism and the philosophy of mind, both in *Mind and Cognition*, edited by G.W. Lycan (Oxford: Blackwell Scientific 1992, pp. 224–51 and 252–74 respectively).

3. Thus, it should be noted, the very foundations of our self-awareness are *conditioned* by the language we must, of necessity, use. It is for this reason that we should guard against the corruption of language, since such corruption necessarily limits the breadth and scope of our *self* and of its expression.The use of the language of *biology* to express the nature of the self should be viewed with some disquiet, since its prescriptive nature imposes severe limits on what can be expressed.

4. With more than a nod in the direction of Jacques Derrida, Dennett (1991) has 'translated' this neurological model of competing states of the system directly into a model of competing drafts or texts. Some of these 'drafts' fight their way to conscious expression to form the present narrative centre of gravity (our 'mistaken' notion of self). The continuous *production* of drafts replaces the notion of a *self* or centre (a psychological source) with the *fiction* of a narrative centre of gravity, whose shaky existence is dependent to a large part on the collaboration of others who ascribe to such drafts a coherence and meaningfulness that they do not intrinsically possess. Since we are all, in this conception (sometimes called semiotic materialism), nothing but the drafts we produce, and since such drafts or texts are themselves not intrinsically meaningful, Dennett is dogged by the circularity of his argument, in that some texts and drafts *must have the meaning conferring properties characteristic of the sorts of agent or self whose existence Dennett is actively denying*. Otherwise, Dennett must insist that it is just another text that confers meaning, which is patently absurd.

REFERENCES

Arthur, D., Dowling, J., and Sharkey, R. (1992) *Mental Health Nursing* (London: WB Saunders/Baillière Tindall).

Baumeister, R. (1987) How the self became a problem, a psychological review of historical research, *Journal of Personality and Social Psychology*, **52**: 163–76.

Bruner, J.S. (1986) *Actual Minds, Possible Worlds* (Cambridge: Harvard University Press).

Dennett, D.C. (1991) *Consciousness Explained* (London: Penguin).

Descartes, R. (1970, trans. E. Anscombe, and P.T. Geach) *Philosophical Writings* (London: Thomas Nelson & Son).

Erikson, E.H. (1950) *Childhood and Society* (New York: W.W. Norton).

Flanagan, O. (1994) *Consciousness Reconsidered* (Cambridge, MA: MIT Press).

Foucault, M. (1980, ed. C. Gordon) *Power/Knowledge* (London: Brighton Books).

Freud, S. (1933) *New Introductory Lectures on Psychoanalysis* (London: Hogarth Press).

Freud, S. (1963) *Standard Edition of The Complete Psychological Works, 1953–1974*, vol. 14 (London: Hogarth Press).

Gergen, K.J. and Gergen, M.M. (1988) Narrative and the Self as relationship, *Advances in Experimental Social Psychology*, **21**: 17–56.

Hermans, H.J.M. and Van Gilst, W. (1991) Self narrative and collective myth. An analysis of the narcissus story, *Journal of Behavioural Science*, **23**: 432–49.

Hermans, H.J.M. Kempen, H.J.G. and van Loon, R.J.P. (1992) The dialogical Self: beyond individualism and rationalism, *American Psychologist*, **47**(1): 23–33.

James, W. (1890, reprinted 1950) *The Principles of Psychology*, 2 vols (New York: Dover Press).

Kernberg, O. (1982) Self, ego, affects and drives, *Journal of American Psychoanalytic Association*, **30**: 893–917.

Kohut, H. (1977) *The Restoration of the Self* (Madison, Connecticut: International Universities Press).

Kvale, S. (1992) Post modern psychology: a contradiction in terms? in Kvale, S. (ed.) *Psychology and Post Modernism*, pp. 31–57 (Calfornia: Sage).

Lacan, J. (1966, trans. A. Sheridan 1977) *Ecrits: A Selection* (London: Tavistock Publications).

Lather, P. (1992) Post Modernism and the Human Sciences, in *Psychology and Post Modernism*, Kvale, S. (ed.), pp. 88–110 (London: Sage).

Madison, G.B. (1988) *The Hermeneutics of Postmodernity: Figures and Themes* (Bloomington: Indiana University Press).

Mead, G.H. (1934, ed. Morris C.W. 1968) *Mind, Self and Society* (London: University of Chicago Press).

Morris, C. (1972) *The Discovery of The Individual, 1050–1200* (London: Camelot Press).

Priest, S. (1991) *Theories of the Mind* (Boston: Houghton & Mifflin).

Sampson, E.E. (1985) The debate on individualism: indigenous psychologies of the individual and their role in personal and societal functioning, *American Psychologist*, **43**: 15–22.

Sampson, E.E. (1988) The decentralisation of identity: towards a revised concept of personal and social order, *American Psychologist*, **40**: 1203–11.

Sandel, M. (1982) *Liberalism and the Limits of Justice* (Cambridge: Cambridge University Press).

Sarbin, T.R. (ed.) (1986) *Narrative Psychology, the Storied Nature of Human Conduct* (New York: Praeger).

Sartre, J-P. (1957, trans. F. Williams and R. Kilpatrick) *The Transcendence of the Ego: An Existentialist Theory of Consciousness* (New York: Noonday Press).

Scott, J. (1987) Critical tensions, *Womens Review of Books*, **5**(1): 17–18.

Stuart, G.W. and Sundeen, S.J. (1991) *Principles and Practice of Psychiatric Nursing* (St Louis: Mosby-Year Book).

Suzuki, D.T. (1968) *The Essence of Buddhism* (Kyoto, Japan: Hozokan).

Zijderveld, A. (1974) *The Abstract Society* (London: Penguin).

CHAPTER TEN

The self and compulsory treatment

EDITOR'S INTRODUCTION

This chapter shows how a proper understanding of the concepts of liberty and autonomy is relevant to questions regarding the justification of compulsory treatment in the context of mental health nursing. Philip Ross proposes that the notion of 'rational autonomy' provides a 'locus of unity' for health-care work, that is to say, this provides an explanation of the point and purpose of health-care work. This seems a plausible claim in the light of the view that much health-care work involves fostering and enhancing the rational autonomy of patients and clients.

Philip Ross points out that the conception of health-care work as fostering the autonomy of patients and clients seems radically challenged by compulsory treatment, for this can plausibly be taken to involve the treatment of a person against that person's wishes. Ross, however, argues that compulsory treatment need not be construed as in conflict with the conception of health-care work just described. His claim is, in effect, that in cases of serious mental disorder, compulsory treatment need not be taken to involve infringement of the liberty of the person concerned, given acceptance of the account of liberty he subscribes to (that of 'positive' liberty).

Furthemore, Philip Ross's defence of compulsory treatment takes on an arch critic of such 'treatment', namely Thomas Szasz. Ross argues that Szasz's opposition to compulsory treatment rests upon the presumption that people who might ordinarily be taken as refusing treatment may well, in fact, be doing no such thing. For it to be true that a person is refusing treatment, it has to be the case that the person is 'rationally autonomous'. However, given the criteria of rational autonomy favoured by Ross, this seems not to be the case in a significant number of instances of compulsory treatment. Hence, the apparently deep conflict between the 'locus of unity' for health-care work and compulsory treatment can be shown to be illusory.

Finally, readers might note that the position taken by Philip Ross concerning the nature of a 'self' is in direct conflict with that described and championed in John Dawson's chapter.

The self and compulsory treatment

Philip Ross

The treatment of those deemed to suffer from mental health problems raises special problems for the point and purpose of nursing. The concept of mental illness has been subject to challenge, together with the legitimacy of forcible treatment. This chapter seeks to defend a concept of coercive mental health care as an attempt to restore a person's control over his or her own behaviour, and suggests that such a notion can clearly distance mental health care from charges of being an instrument for the enforcement of behavioural conformity. The connection between this notion and the philosophical notion of 'positive liberty' is noted, together with the limits it places on the kind of coercive care offered and who is deemed a fit subject for such care.

I begin this chapter by stating what might appear to be obvious: nursing, in common with some other professions, is concerned with helping people; nursing is a caring profession. Clarke (1991, p. 39) suggests that such a generalised definition of the business of nursing might imply that 'there is no such 'thing' as nursing, no uniqueness in the mix but, instead, a mix of different therapeutic activities, often directed towards qualitatively different ends'. Where is the 'locus of unity', he asks, even within the ambit of psychiatric nursing, never mind nursing generally? I hope to propose that there may be a 'locus of unity' and that this centres on a specific conception of health and thus generates the point and purpose of health care. The proposed conception of the point and purpose of health care, put briefly, is the restoration and/or enhancement of (rational) autonomy. I suggest, furthermore, that this constitutes a single qualitative end and that it is equally applicable in the treatment of broken limbs as it is mental disorders.

It should be obvious that the proposed candidate for the 'locus of unity' extends beyond nursing and ought to be shared by other health-care professionals. My focus, however, is restricted to psychiatry and to the problem of forcible treatment. This represents, at least superficially, the greatest challenge to respect for autonomy and to a conception of health care centred on the project of the enhancement of the autonomy of patients and clients.

NEGATIVE AND POSITIVE LIBERTY

The use of force presents an ethical problem in so far as it is regarded as incompatible with respect for individual freedom or autonomy. As Berlin writes, in his classic study of individual liberty, '[To] coerce a man is to deprive him of freedom' (1969, p. 121). This, as he notes, conflicts with the standard *negative* view of individual freedom in which:

> I am normally said to be free to the degree to which no man interferes with my activity.... . If I am prevented by others from doing what I could otherwise do, I am to that degree unfree.... . (Berlin, 1969, p. 122)

There is, however, another concept of freedom, which Berlin calls '*positive* liberty where the positive sense of the word "liberty" derives from the wish on the part of the individual to be his own master' (1969, p. 131). The difference between the negative and positive conceptions of liberty is usually seen in terms of the difference between 'freedom from' and 'freedom to', the former corresponding to the negative conception and the latter to the positive. I intend, in this chapter to defend the positive conception of liberty.

THE CONCEPT OF MENTAL ILLNESS: THE CRITIQUE
OF THOMAS SZASZ

The reader might be forgiven at this point for wondering what a philosophical debate concerning the proper definition of liberty has to do with the subject of mental health and coercive or forcible psychiatric care. Psychiatry, especially coercive or forcible psychiatric intervention, has come under more or less sustained attack from various quarters over the past three decades. Indeed, these critics have acquired a label: the *anti-psychiatry movement*. Foremost among the anti-psychiatrists, arguably, is (paradoxically) the psychiatrist Thomas Szasz.

The description of Szasz as an anti-psychiatrist needs qualifying. He is not opposed to the practice of psychiatry as such. Rather, the focus of his opposition is what he terms the 'bureaucratic system of institutional psychiatry and its concentration camps called "mental hospitals"' (Szasz, 1974, p. 6). Forcible psychiatric intervention or commitment, the detention of persons deemed to be suffering mental disorder and their treatment against their will, is, according to Szsaz, an integral part of 'institutional psychiatry' and is, he insists, a 'crime against humanity', a 'crass violation of contemporary concepts of fundamental human rights' (1974, p. 112).

Central to Szasz's attack on institutional psychiatry is his critique of the concept of mental illness itself. The concept of mental illness, Szasz insists, is a myth. It is worth noting that mental illness is not defined in UK legislation (Mason and McCall Smith, 1994, p. 396). The root of the conceptual problem of mental illness arises from confusion regarding the notion of *mind*. If by the concept of mind (and thus diseases or illnesses of the mind) is meant the brain, and thus diseases or illnesses of the brain, the conceptual problem disappears. Yet, if mental illness means brain disease, the concept of mental illness is redundant. Mental illness is reduced to disease of a bodily organ: the brain (Szasz, 1982).

Yet, Szasz argues, this is not what is meant by mental illness, nor, philosophically speaking, could it be:

> [When] we speak of physical disturbances, we mean either signs (for example, a fever) or symptoms (for example, pain). We speak of mental symptoms, on the other hand, when we refer to a patient's *communications about himself, others, and the world about him...* the statement that 'X is a mental symptom' involves rendering a judgment. (Szasz, 1982, pp. 20–1)

What judgment is this?: essentially a 'covert comparison or matching of the patient's ideas, concepts or beliefs with those of the observer and the society in which they live' (Szasz, 1982, p. 21). In other words, the labelling of a person as mentally ill is not a statement about that person's brain states but rather a judgement about the person's behaviour. The behaviour or beliefs of the person labelled *patient* are being contrasted with those of the psychiatrist, the therapeutic community and the wider society. The behaviour is judged 'abnormal' by this standard of comparison, and the object of treatment is to correct those beliefs or behaviour and substitute for them beliefs or behaviours that the community regards as 'normal'. This point applies, Szasz argues, even in the case of those patients who suffer from 'demonstrable diseases of the brain' (Szasz, 1974, p. 114). He cites as examples individuals intoxicated with alcohol or other drugs, or elderly people suffering from degenerative diseases of the brain:

> [When] patients with demonstrable diseases of the brain are involuntarily hospitalized, the primary purpose is to exercise social control over their behaviour. (Szasz, 1974, p. 114)

This concept of 'social control' (Szasz, 1974) is crucial for Szasz. The concept of illness, he argues, 'whether bodily or mental, implies *deviation from some clearly defined norm*' (Szasz, 1982, p. 21). In the case of physical illness, the norm is the 'structural and functional integrity of the human body', but in the case of mental illness, the norm can only be defined in terms of '*psychosocial, ethical* and *legal* concepts' (Szasz, 1982, p. 21). Psychiatric diagnoses, Szasz argues, 'do not point to anatomical or physiological lesions and do not suggest causal agents, but allude only to human behaviours' (1991, p. 1576). Forcible psychiatric intervention, in this line of argument, amounts to the imposition of behavioural norms.

What exactly, then, does Szasz recommend in place of institutional psychiatry? The conduct of human beings, he argues, 'is always rule-following, strategic and meaningful' (Szasz, 1972, pp. 275–6). Human relations should be analysed 'as if they were games, the behaviour of the players being governed by explicit or tacit game rules' (Szasz, 1972, pp. 275–6). In most cases of *voluntary* psychotherapy, the therapist 'tries to elucidate the inexplicit game rules by which the client conducts himself; and to help the client scrutinize the goals and values of the life games he plays' (Szasz, 1972, pp. 275–6). Voluntary psychiatric treatment does not violate the concept of self-ownership, the idea that a person owns his or her own body. This notion goes back at least as far as the 17th-century English philosopher John Locke (1690, 1924, ch. v, para. 27). Also, it is the cornerstone of the libertarian political philosophy of, for example, Robert Nozick (1974). Szasz argues that, in free societies:

> [The] relationship between physician and patient is predicated on the legal presumption that the individual 'owns' his body and his personality. (Szasz, 1974, p. 115)

Involuntary psychiatric intervention is an invasion of privacy, a violation of private property rights, the property rights one has in one's own person. Voluntary psychiatric intervention, on the Szaszian model, however, is predicated on the recognition that psychiatry deals in 'problems in living', that mental illness is a name for 'problems in living' (Szasz, 1982). The therapist attempts to elucidate the rules by which the client conducts him or herself and presumably to help clients re-orient their behaviour or their lives if that is what they so wish.

Institutional psychiatry is replaced, in Szasz's psychiatric prescription, by the free, contractual relationship between therapist and client. Szasz asks, is the 'guiding value of psychiatry individualism or collectivism?... Does psychiatry aspire to be the servant of the individual or of the state?' (Szasz, 1974, p. 10). The implication is, of course, that institutional psychiatry, masking itself behind the pseudo-science of 'mental illness', is in the service of the collective, the state, community or society. Institutional psychiatry is an instrument for maintaining behavioural conformity at the expense of individual freedom. Voluntary, contractual psychotherapy, on the other hand, champions the individual and respects the individual integrity and dignity that self-ownership confers.

MENTAL HEALTH AS RATIONAL AUTONOMY

Szasz's critique of what he terms 'institutional psychiatry' is well known. The above is intended only as a summary. The point, however, is how to respond to Szasz'z challenge. It is hardly adequate to say 'despite the lack of clarity in the term, most people regard mental illness as a fact' (Chadwick and Tadd, 1992, p. 112). Most people might be wrong. It is, however, for my purposes, important to note that, in dismissing mental illness as a myth, 'people who are really very ill might be denied treatment' (Chadwick and Tadd, 1992, p. 112). What is required is a conceptual analysis that disputes Szasz's identification of mental illness with 'problems in living' and a defence of coercive psychiatric interventions in the name of a clarified conception of mental health.

It will be suggested here that Edwards (1982) has the essence of the matter. He conceives of mental health as 'rational autonomy'. Correspondingly, 'mental illness' means only those 'undesirable mental/behavioural deviations which involve primarily an extreme and prolonged inability to know and deal in a rational and autonomous way with oneself and one's social and physical environment' (Edwards, 1982, p. 70). Edwards refers to his conception of mental health as a conservative one that effectively resists the tendency towards the medicalisation of life (Illich, 1976), in which all human problems are reduced to medical or pseudo-medical ones.

The attraction of Edwards' conception, it seems to me, consists in its potential for rescuing the reputation of psychiatry and, indeed, I would argue, forcible psychiatric intervention. The idea of mental health as rational autonomy seems to me to imply that the object of psychiatry, including compulsory treatment, is not to force the non-conforming to conform but rather to enable those who have lost control over their own behaviour (and indeed their own lives) to regain that control. The issue is not the behaviour of the person labelled 'mentally ill' as such, but rather whether that person is in control of his or her own behaviour. Is the person concerned, in Edwards' phrase, 'freely actualizing a capacity for making [their] own choices' (1982, p. 71)?

Other authors have a similar conception of mental health and of mental illness, as Edwards notes. Thus, Engelhardt (1982) argues that the 'goals of psychotherapy are similar to those of medicine in general... . Both seek to remove hindrances and augment a patient's freedom' (1982, p. 61). Psychotherapy, he argues, aims at 'getting one to value reality' and at 'freeing one from drives and forces that encumber free action'; it is 'directed toward liberating the patient from the control of unconscious drives and unacknowledged forces' (1982, p. 62), a notion of the goal of psychotherapy that he, unsurprisingly, argues is 'consonant with themes' in the work of the figure most closely associated in the public mind with psychoanalysis – Sigmund Freud (Engelhardt, 1982, p. 61).

The conception of mental health and mental illness just canvassed seems also to underlie Fulford's discussion of the concept of a disease (1993). Whereas, Fulford argues, in physical medicine, failure of function is important and is regarded as the 'root concept', in psychiatry 'the concept of *failure of action*, though not always recognizable for what it is, is, in many contexts, at least as prominent as that of failure of function' (Fulford, 1993, p. 89). He gives examples from the World Health Organization's *International Classification of Diseases*:

> the hysterical neurotic is distinguished from the malingerer by his symptoms not being intentional; the addict has 'lost control' of his use of drugs or alcohol; and the obsessional is unable to resist senselessly repeating his actions. (Fulford, 1993, p. 89)

Failure of action, Fulford suggests, is and should be the 'root concept' in psychiatry and thus in mental health and illness. The implication of Fulford's analysis reinforces the notion in Edwards and Engelhardt that the function of psychiatric intervention is to promote autonomy or freedom of action. If mental illness is to be understood principally in terms of failure of action, the object of psychiatric care ought to be to restore the client or patient's capacity for (free) action. Indeed, this notion of mental health as rational autonomy seems to underpin the general public's ascription of health and illness, or what Holmes calls '"lay" theories of illness':

empirical evidence consistently identifies self-determination, self-control and freedom from mental conflict as major components of lay conceptions of health. (1991, p. 81)

Of course, current UK legislation excludes alcoholism and drug addiction from being categorised as mental disorders for the purposes of admission (Mason and McCall Smith, 1994, p. 395). However, one could argue, consistent with the idea of mental health as rational autonomy, that alcoholics and drug addicts are still in a position to choose to overcome their addictions if they wish to do so.

IS RATIONAL AUTONOMY ITSELF A BEHAVIOURAL STANDARD?

Psychotherapy, Engelhardt argues, 'involves one in a question of values, but not in a particular ethic' (1982, p. 62). Psychotherapy, in advancing freedom or autonomy, Engelhardt argues, is not advancing an ethic as such but rather a meta-ethic. The technical philosophical phrase 'meta-ethics' needs explaining. Ethics, as such, is concerned with first-order questions: how ought one to conduct oneself generally or in a given situation. Meta-ethics, on the other hand, is concerned with second-order questions such as 'What does it mean to say that one ought to do x?'; 'Can one know that a course of action is morally wrong in the same way that we claim to know that the earth is not flat?' How does Engelhardt make use of this notion of meta-ethics?:

A possible meta-ethical proposition would be, 'ethics involves a choice between goods or duties and, therefore, involves the general value of responsible choice or *free* choice. (1982, p. 62)

However, I am unconvinced by this philosophical move. If freedom or autonomy is valuable, this must refer to some ethic whereby freedom is regarded as valuable. Meta-ethics does not concern itself with what is or is not of value; it concerns itself, amongst other things, with the meaning of the word 'valuable'. In the case of the client or patient deemed to be mentally ill and, in Engelhardt's definition, disabled by unconscious and unacknowledged forces, it is always open to those engaged in providing care and treatment to conclude that they have no business in rescuing the person concerned from their psychological disablement. If those providing care or society conclude otherwise, it means that freedom is valued over 'unfreedom' so to speak.

The real issue, however, and the substance of Engelhardt's thesis, is whether advancing freedom or autonomy involves getting patients or clients to adopt a prescribed mode of behaving. If it does, suspicions again arise that psychiatric intervention is merely a procedure for enforcing behavioural conformity and for eliminating behaviour regarded as deviant. Is 'setting the stage for the possibility of ethical decisions' or 'integrating [a patient's] mental life so that he can come to effective terms with his impulses and his external environment' (Engelhardt, 1982, p. 62) advancing a socially prescribed way of behaving?

The same question arises in regard to Edwards's conception of rational autonomy. It involves, according to Edwards, 'actualizing a capacity for making one's own choices, managing one's own practical affairs and assuming responsibility for one's own life, its station and its duties' (1982, p. 71). Actualising a capacity for making one's own choices seems to be reasonably neutral in so far as enabling people to make their own choices does not entail forcing them to make certain prescribed choices. One could, for example, freely choose to engage in 'deviant' behaviour. What follows, however, takes one beyond the notion of freely made choices. In particular, the reference to taking responsibility for one's station and its duties could imply behavioural prescription. How does one deal, for example, with the patient or client who freely rejects his or her station and its duties?

Similar problems can occur with the notion of rationality; Edwards lists seven points in his philosophical explication of it. The list includes the ability to distinguish means from ends and to identify means likely to lead to the realisation of 'consciously envisioned goals' (1982, p. 72), thinking logically, having factual beliefs that are supported by adequate empirical evidence, being able to give reasons for one's behaviour/beliefs and having values that have been 'adopted under conditions of freedom, enlightenment, and impartiality' (1982, p. 72). This seems to me to be, potentially, a rather expansive interpretation of the idea, in contrast to Edwards' stated 'conservative' conception of mental illness. A bigot may have not have chosen her or his values under conditions of impartiality, the same might be said of a fanatic, but I would be disinclined to call such persons mentally ill. Equally, an inability to think logically would not surely incline us to ascribe mental illness (although Edwards does talk here of extreme and persistent illogicality and irrationality).

The concept of rationality is the subject of an extensive philosophical literature. The celebrated English philosopher Bertrand Russell (1872–1970) defines it thus:

'Reason' has a perfectly clear and precise meaning. It signifies the choice of the right means to an end that you wish to achieve. It has nothing whatever to do with the choice of ends. (1954, p. 8)

This notion of rationality can be characterised as a purely instrumental conception. It centres only on means to ends and does not extend to consideration of the rationality or otherwise of the chosen ends themselves. How would the instrumental conception work in practice with regard to those deemed to be mentally ill? Graham (1993, p. 113) cites a case that is useful in this regard. This involved a man who thought he had two heads. One of the heads, the alien head, taunted him with hostile thoughts. The man's solution to this predicament was to attempt to shoot his alien head off with a revolver. Graham notes that the man survived but was seriously wounded and died some 2 years later from chronic infection caused by the shooting. Was this a rational action and should one deem the person concerned rationally autonomous?: Graham himself defines rational action as 'behaviour done for reasons or purposes of the agent' (1993, p. 109).

On Graham's account of rationality, and indeed on Russell's instrumental conception, one would have to conclude that the person concerned is rational. He is also autonomous: he appears to have been actualising a capacity for making his own choices. As Graham notes, in the case cited, the man was acting for a reason: furthermore, he was acting from a 'subjectively good reason' (1993, p. 113). In terms of the man's own perception of his predicament, one might conclude that he had good reason to act the way he did. Yet, Graham argues, this action was rational only internally (from the agent's perspective) but not externally (from the third-person perspective). He concludes:

The shooting was externally irrational on two grounds. First, it stemmed from a grossly unhealthy or imprudent desire. The desire to shoot ticketed him for disaster. Second, it rested on a belief (that he had two heads) which was not merely false but plainly false and should have been false to the man. (1993, p. 113)

A difficulty here, arising from Graham's conclusion, is that one may be in danger of so fleshing out one's conception of rationality (as in the case of Edwards's conception of autonomy) that one smuggles in societal norms. In other words, the project to eliminate deviant behaviour in the name of psychiatry has resurrected itself in the guise of the pursuit of rational autonomy, thereby giving rise to the very thing anti-psychiatrists, such as Szasz, object to. Nozick (1993, p. 176) is in favour of a conception of rationality that is broader than the instrumental conception. The rational person, he argues, is not merely the person who chooses the best means of satisfying his or her goals or desires but the person whose goals and desires are arrived at in a rational way and who has rational beliefs:

> The rationality of a belief or action is a matter of its responsiveness to the reasons for and against, and of the process by which those reasons are generated. (Nozick, 1993, p. 107)

This interpretation is also adopted by Elster. For him, rationality includes 'forming the best-grounded belief, for given evidence; and collecting the right amount of evidence for given desires and... beliefs' (1990, p. 21). Nozick is aware of the potential dangers inherent in this substantive conception of rationality. He warns that a:

> fully specified theory of substantive rationality opens the door to despotic requirements, externally imposed... . Instrumental rationality leaves us the room to pursue our *own* goals autonomously. (1993, p. 176)

In other words, in a substantive conception of rationality, one is in danger of imposing goals, beliefs and modes of behaviour on mentally ill clients rather than enabling them to form their own beliefs and desires and pursue their own goals. Consider again the case cited by Graham. As a way out of this problem, one might conclude that this individual would not have acted as he did had he not falsely believed that he had two heads and would not have attempted to shoot his 'alien head' if he had realised the real danger to himself. Hypothetically speaking, had this individual come to the attention of mental health services prior to his attempt to destroy his 'alien head', one might have been justified in compulsorily treating him. This might have been done in order to rescue him from his delusions, and to restore him to those beliefs and that mode of behaviour that he would have adopted but for the particular mental illness from which he was suffering.

The problems with such views are similar to the controversy surrounding the notion of positive liberty. According to Berlin, with the positive conception of liberty:

> I am in a position to ignore the actual wishes of men... to... oppress... them in the name... of [their] 'true', albeit often submerged and inarticulate, [selves]. (1969, p. 133)

Positive liberty enables one to posit a 'true' self with true desires and wishes and goals behind the false self with its false desires, wishes and goals. Positive liberty provides for a situation in which, in Rousseau's famous phrase, persons can be 'forced to be free' (1762, I, ch. vii, p. 177).

Berlin's analysis has been challenged by Taylor (1986). The negative liberty that Berlin champions, which focuses only on the absence of external obstacles to a person's pursuing his or her own goals, is, Taylor argues, too narrow. It ignores internal obstacles to pursuing one's own goals. The 'internally fettered man', Taylor argues, 'is not free' (p. 110). One could conceivably argue that persons suffering from what are judged to be delusional states are internally fettered and thus not free or autonomous.

Rational autonomy, then, I conclude, consists in actualising a capacity for making one's own choices and, in Nozick's phrase, being 'responsive to the reasons for and against' (1993, p. 107) beliefs and courses of action. Construed as such, rational autonomy is free of the taint of social control and behavioural or ideological conformity. Sanity is defined not in terms of a person's beliefs, whether empirical or evaluative, nor in terms of the way a person behaves; it is concerned with how a person arrives at his or her beliefs and desires and whether a person is capable of freely acting on those beliefs and desires.

Of course, the only evidence one could have for rational autonomy is behavioural; it is not an explicit reference to the workings of the mind or the brain. However, questioning a person's reasons for acting in a certain way or having a certain belief is not itself to question those beliefs or those actions. One final point in this section: one could argue that a fanatic is not responsive to reasons for and against particular actions or beliefs. I suggest, however, that the fanatic *chooses* to be closed to rational considerations.

RATIONAL AUTONOMY AND THE CONCEPTION OF THE SELF

Does the definition of mental health as rational autonomy imply a certain philosophy of mind? In defining mental health as rational autonomy, one is not committing oneself to any particular theory of the *source* or *cause* of the absence of rational autonomy in a patient or client. Nurses who promote the idea or aim of enhancing or promoting rational autonomy are not, therefore, trespassing into the murky controversy between, for example, behaviourists and non-behaviourists in psychology and psychiatry. The issue here is not what the cause of mental illness is but what it is to restore a person to mental health. Of course, the theory one adopts to explain the mental illness will affect the treatment prescribed, but whatever treatment is prescribed, the aim or objective of treatment should remain unchanged.

One particular view to which the concept of rational autonomy must logically be committed, however, is the notion that a person can control his or her behaviour. Restoring a person's control over personal behaviour logically implies that persons control or can control their own behaviour, that human behaviour issues, at least in part, from human will, decision or choice. This, in turn, seems to presuppose a view of the mind and the relationship between mind and body associated with the French 17th-century philosopher Descartes (1641); it is a philosophy of mind that has come under sustained attack from philosophers of mind in the 20th century.

Actualising a capacity for making one's own choices seems logically to imply that choices are made by the person that are prior to action and where action issues as a result of the choices or decisions made. Of course, it is still possible to claim that those choices or decisions are themselves determined by social or genetic influences, yet one is implicitly positing a connection between mental decision and bodily action, the 'rational self' controlling behaviour.

Dennett (1991, p. 424) refers to this conception of self as the 'simplistic Boss of the Body, Ghost in the Machine... model'. The notion of the ghost in the machine is a pejorative phrase used by the philosopher Gilbert Ryle (1963, p. 17) to dismiss Descartes' dualist philosophy of mind. The essence of Cartesian dualism is the separation of mind and body, where the mind or the soul or the self is nonphysical and controls the body, which obviously is physical. Thus, the mind, 'self' or 'ego' appears in Descartes' philosophy as the non-physical controller of a person's actions. Among the many questions Ryle raises, one concerns just how a non-physical mind/self/soul can control the physical body. How does a non-physical thing connect with a physical thing? He also dismisses the view of the mind as a 'thing' as a 'category mistake'.

Dennett similarly argues that 'selves are not independently existing soul-pearls' (1991, p. 423), the bosses of their respective bodies. Just what is a self, then, according to Dennett? It is, he argues, a 'centre of narrative gravity', a 'magnificent fiction', but a necessary fiction (1991, p. 429). The self is an abstraction, a necessary presupposition, Humphrey and Dennett argue (1991). Human beings create, via their imaginations, one or more selves. The dominant, or best-supported, self becomes something like a 'head of mind'. This conception of the human self, Humphrey and Dennett (1991) argue, is consistent with evidence from biology and artificial intelligence.

However, as Glover notes:

The thought that what someone does is a product of sub-systems (independent centres of control within the person) conflicts with our ordinary ideas about the unity of a person and about our awareness of our own mind. (1989, p. 25)

Many of Humphrey and Dennett's conclusions derive from studies on persons with multiple personality disorder. There is also, however, the phenomenon of 'split-brain' patients (see Nagel, 1976); these are people in whom the corpus callosum (the structure that connects the two cerebral hemispheres) has been severed (an operation carried out in the course of treatment for epilepsy). Both these conditions seem to undermine the 'single self', 'boss of the body' conception of the human person.

If rational autonomy implies the notion of a rational self in control of that self's behaviour, is the pursuit of rational autonomy the pursuit of a fiction? I would argue that we distinguish between actions and events in which the language of action is logically different from the language of events (Davidson, 1976). As Graham explains:

rational action is performed for a reason, whereas mere movement happens because of a cause. Equivalently: every rational action is explained by reference to the agent's reason for doing it, whereas movements are explained by reference to causes. (1993, p. 110)

There is a long-standing philosophical debate concerning whether reasons are causes and, if so, what kinds of cause, which I have not the space to go into here. However, I agree with Graham and with Ginet. As the latter puts it, while it may not be necessary for actions to have explanations in terms of the agent's motives, in the 'light of conceptual connections that do obtain... a complete account of the nature of action should include an account of that sort of explanation' (1990, p. 4). Similarly, the notion of free action is not easily dispensed with. For Skinner (1973), the notion of 'autonomous man' is a pre-scientific notion that will in time be superseded by a science of human behaviour in which human action is seen to be the result of environmental and genetic conditioning. Yet Skinner's social proposals, the use of a 'technology of human behaviour' to eliminate criminality, for example, presuppose the concept of free will. Someone must operate the technology of human behaviour to consciously chosen goals. Deciding which values, goals or policies to adopt logically presupposes freedom.

If the self is merely a 'centre of narrative gravity', rational autonomy may merely consist in enabling persons to see themselves in such a way, to be able to conceive of a narrative or story that rationally integrates their biography without implying that they are in charge of it. It would seem to me, however, that the idea of choice without a chooser is at the very least linguistically problematical.

CONCLUSION

In response to Szasz's question 'Does psychiatry wish to serve the state or the individual?', I think the correct answer is 'Both'. Psychiatric interventions should aim to enhance or restore a person's rational autonomy. It is only the latter, in my view, that justifies compulsory treatment. The issue as regards forcible psychiatric intervention is not whether persons are a threat to themselves or to others; these are not health matters at all. The question is whether a person's behaviour is rationally integrated. Is such persons' behaviour an expression of their own reasonings and choices, and are they responsive to reasons? Mere freedom from coercion (negative liberty) is morally empty. One is inclined to ask with Plant (1991, p. 244), just what is so valuable about freedom from coercion? If the answer is so that persons can live their lives in their own way, mere freedom from interference or coercion may not suffice. There may be external obstacles to realising one's own choices (lack of access to material resources, for example). There may also be *internal* obstacles, for example, mental illness on the definition adopted in this chapter.

I suggested that psychiatry may be in the service also of the state or community. The just society is, in my view, one that provides for active participation by the citizens of the state or community. There is no room to expand on this matter here, but active participation in the life of the community requires rational autonomy. As Sedgwick (1982) notes, Szasz's attack on 'institutional psychiatry' coincides with a general attack on what might be called the welfare or public service state. The state's activities, according to the prevailing political philosophy in the United Kingdom and the United States particularly in the 1980s, should be minimal, what Nozick calls the 'minimal state' (1974, p. ix), confined, in his view, to protecting persons from force, fraud and theft and enforcing contracts. There is no moral justification, Nozick argues, for forcing some persons to aid others or for prohibiting activities to people for their own good or protection. Anti-welfare goes hand in hand with anti-paternalism.

Respect for meaningful freedom and active citizenship (I will leave aside the debate about justice in the distribution of material resources), I would argue, requires more than a minimal state. It requires, amongst other things, provision for a public mental health service to cater for those persons unfortunate enough to lose their rational autonomy. Paradoxically, paternalism *can* be justified in the name of restoring freedom or autonomy. The removal of internal psychological obstacles to freedom or autonomy may be a way of justifying the temporary use of force.

The psychiatric nurse should, I suggest, be an advocate for autonomy. The idea of nurse advocacy has come under attack for its ambiguity from some commentators (Melia, 1989). Does advocacy mean standing up for patients' best interests or the right of patients to make their own choices and decisions? I would argue that autonomy is the core concept but that this need not rule out cooperating in the forcible treatment of patients who evidence a radical breakdown in their capacity for rational autonomy. Again, standing up for rational autonomy does not imply commitment to any particular theory of the nature or cause of specific mental illnesses, or indeed their treatment. Rational autonomy, and thus advocacy for rational autonomy, is *folk psychological*. As Holdsworth (1995, p. 479) notes, folk psychology 'expresses in ordinary language the phenomena any scientific theory seeks to explain'; it 'explains behaviour by reference to purposes rather then antecedent causes' (p. 478). It thus fits in neatly with Graham's concept of rational action (1993). It also escapes the controversy surrounding competing psychological and psychiatric schools in which, according to Tyrer and Steinberg (1993, p. 1), there is 'no indication that psychiatry has a common theoretical base'.

In conclusion, it has been argued above that freedom is 'self-directedness'. The capacity for self-directedness can be compromised by mental health problems. The temporary use of force can be morally justified in the name of restoring a person's capacity for self-directedness or rational autonomy, where mental health is defined in terms of rational autonomy. Rational autonomy is the basis for the folk-psychological view of the human person. Finally, rational autonomy is necessary for active citizenship. Societies ought, therefore, to provide publicly funded mental health services.

REFERENCES

Berlin, I. (1969) *Four Essays on Liberty* (Oxford: Oxford University Press).
Chadwick, R. and Tadd, W. (1992) *Ethics and Nursing Practice* (Basingstoke: Macmillan).
Clarke, L. (1991) Ideological themes in mental health nursing, in Barker, P.J. and Baldwin, S. (eds) *Ethical Issues in Mental Health*, pp. 27–46 (London: Chapman & Hall).
Davidson, D. (1976) Psychology as philosophy, in Glover, J. (ed.) *The Philosophy of Mind*, pp. 101–10 (Oxford: Oxford University Press).
Dennett, D.C. (1991) *Consciousness Explained* (Middlesex: Penguin).
Descartes, R. (1641, trans. F.E. Sutcliffe, 1968) *Discourse on Method and the Meditations* (Middlesex: Penguin).
Edwards, R.B. (1982) Mental health as rational autonomy, in Edwards, R.B. (ed.) *Psychiatry and Ethics*, pp. 68–78 (New York: Prometheus).
Elster, J. (1990) When rationality fails, in Cook, K.S. and Levi, M. (eds) *The Limits of Rationality*, pp. 19–46 (Chicago: University of Chicago Press).
Engelhardt, H. Jr (1982) Psychotherapy as Meta-ethics, in Edwards, R.B. (ed.) *Psychiatry and Ethics*, pp. 61–7 (New York: Prometheus).
Fulford, K.W.M. (1993) The concept of a disease, in Bloch, S. and Chodoff, P. (eds) *Psychiatric Ethics*, pp. 77–100 (Oxford: Oxford University Press).
Ginet, C. (1990) *On Action* (Cambridge: Cambridge University Press).
Glover, J. (1989) *I: The Philosophy and Psychology of Personal Identity* (Middlesex: Penguin).
Graham, G. (1993) *Philosophy of Mind: An Introduction* (Oxford: Blackwell).
Holdsworth, N. (1995) From psychiatric science to folk psychology: an ordinary language model for mental health nurses, *Journal of Advanced Nursing*, **21**: 476–86.
Holmes, C. (1991) Psychopathic disorder: a category mistake?, *Journal of Medical Ethics*, **17**: 77–85.
Humphrey, N. and Dennett, D.C. (1991) Speaking for ourselves: an assessment of multiple personality disorder, in Kolak, D. and Martin, R. (eds) *Self and Identity: Contemporary Philosophical Issues*, pp. 144–62 (New York: Macmillan).
Illich, I. (1976) *Medical Nemesis: The Expropriation of Health* (New York: Pantheon).
Locke, J. (first published 1690, 1924, reprinted 1960) *Two Treatises of Government* (New York: Everyman).
Mason, J.K. and McCall Smith, R.A. (1994) *Law and Medical Ethics*, 4th edn (London: Butterworth).
Melia, K. (1989) *Everyday Nursing Ethics* (Basingstoke: Macmillan).
Mill, J.S. (1859, ed. G. Himmelfarb 1974) *On Liberty* (Middlesex: Penguin).
Nagel, T. (1976) Brain bisection and the unity of consciousness, in Glover, J. (ed.) *The Philosophy of Mind*, pp. 111–25 (Oxford: Oxford University Press).
Nozick, R. (1974) *Anarchy, State and Utopia* (Oxford: Blackwell).
Nozick, R. (1993) *The Nature of Rationality* (Princeton: Princeton University Press).

Parfit, D. (1987) Divided minds and the nature of persons, in Blakemore C. and Greenfield, S. (eds) *Mindwaves: Thoughts on Intelligence, Identity and Consciousness*, pp. 19–26 (Oxford: Blackwell).

Plant, R. (1991) *Modern Political Thought* (Oxford: Blackwell).

Rousseau, J.J (1762) The social contract, in Cole, G.D.H. (1973) *The Social Contract and Discourses* (London: Dent).

Russell, B. (1954) *Human Society in Ethics and Politics* (London: Allen & Unwin).

Ryle, G. (1963) *The Concept Of Mind* (Middlesex: Peregrine).

Sedgwick, P. (1982) *Psycho Politics* (London: Pluto).

Skinner, B.F. (1973) *Beyond Freedom and Dignity* (Middlesex: Penguin).

Szasz, T.S. (1972) *The Myth of Mental Illness* (St Albans: Paladin).

Szasz, T.S. (1974) *Ideology and Insanity* (Middlesex: Penguin).

Szasz, T.S. (1982) The myth of mental illness, in Edwards, R.B. (ed.) *Psychiatry and Ethics*, pp. 19–28 (New York: Prometheus).

Szasz, T.S. (1991) Diagnoses are not diseases, *The Lancet*, **338**, 1574–6.

Taylor, C. (1986) What's wrong with negative liberty?, in Stewart, R.M. (ed.) *Readings in Social and Political Philosophy*, pp. 100–12 (New York: Oxford University Press).

Tyrer, P and Steinberg, D. (1993) *Models for Mental Disorder: Conceptual Models in Psychiatry* (Chichester: John Wiley).

Made in the USA
Middletown, DE
14 September 2017